"This is a masterwork in Creative Arts Therapies by a seasoned artist/therapist. As a Jungian-oriented drama therapist, who has spent many years working with myth and fairy tale, myself, I cannot recommend this book highly enough. It inspires, guides and educates. What a gift for the next generation!"

—Stephen Snow, Ph.D., RDT-BCT,
Professor of Drama Therapy, Co-founder of Graduate
Drama Therapy Program, Concordia University

"*The Story Within* is a passport to the deep places in us. Yehudit Silverman speaks equally to seekers, therapists, and artists of all mediums. Yehudit's own story, La Loba, is a generous through line, teaching us how story moves us and moves in us, weaving the golden threads of the archetypal realm into our contemporary lives to find meaning, resolve conflict and heal trauma."

—Pat B. Allen, Ph.D., ATR, Author of Art is a way
of knowing *and* Art is a spiritual path

"This book invites us on a journey through the landscapes of the deeply personal and the profoundly collective. Our guide is patient, steadfast and wise in her offering of transformation through creative arts. Personally, my experience with the *Story Within* has had an enormous impact on my education, my clinical trajectory and more recently my work as a trauma therapist—this is a valuable resource for anyone dedicated to the transformation and alleviation of human suffering."

—Dr. Kate Drury, Clinical Psychologist, Trauma-focused
Therapy Program at the Jewish General Hospital

The Story Within

of related interest

Improvisation in the Expressive and Performing Arts
The Relationship between Shaping and Letting-go
Beliz Demircioglu
Foreword by Stephen K. Levine
ISBN 978 1 78592 575 7
eISBN 978 1 78450 979 8

Collaborations Within and Between Dramatherapy and Music Therapy
Experiences, Challenges and Opportunities in Clinical and Training Contexts
Edited by Amelia Oldfield and Mandy Carr
Foreword by Rebecca Applin Warner
ISBN 978 1 78592 135 3
eISBN 978 1 78450 402 1

New Developments in Expressive Arts Therapy
The Play of Poiesis
Edited by Ellen G. Levine and Stephen K. Levine
ISBN 978 1 78592 247 3
eISBN 978 1 78450 532 5

Empowering Therapeutic Practice
Integrating Psychodrama into other Therapies
Edited by Paul Holmes, Mark Farrall and Kate Kirk
ISBN 978 1 84905 458 4
eISBN 978 0 85700 834 3

Dramatherapy with Myth and Fairytale
The Golden Stories of Sesame
Jenny Pearson, Mary Smail and Pat Watts
Illustrated by Camilla Jessel
ISBN 978 1 84905 030 2
eISBN 978 0 85700 438 3

THE STORY WITHIN

Myth and Fairy Tale in Therapy

Yehudit Silverman

Foreword by Phil Jones

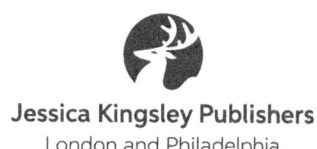

Jessica Kingsley Publishers
London and Philadelphia

First published in 2020
by Jessica Kingsley Publishers
73 Collier Street
London N1 9BE, UK
and
400 Market Street, Suite 400
Philadelphia, PA 19106, USA

www.jkp.com

Copyright © Yehudit Silverman 2020
Foreword copyright © Phil Jones 2020

Front cover image source: mask created by Yehudit Silverman.

All photographs are taken from Silverman, Y. (2004). *The Story Within—Myth and Fairy Tale in Therapy* (documentary film).

All rights reserved. No part of this publication may be reproduced in any material form (including photocopying, storing in any medium by electronic means or transmitting) without the written permission of the copyright owner except in accordance with the provisions of the law or under terms of a licence issued in the UK by the Copyright Licensing Agency Ltd. www.cla.co.uk or in overseas territories by the relevant reproduction rights organisation, for details see www.ifrro.org. Applications for the copyright owner's written permission to reproduce any part of this publication should be addressed to the publisher.

Warning: The doing of an unauthorised act in relation to a copyright work may result in both a civil claim for damages and criminal prosecution.

Library of Congress Cataloging in Publication Data
A CIP catalog record for this book is available from the Library of Congress

British Library Cataloguing in Publication Data
A CIP catalogue record for this book is available from the British Library

ISBN 978 1 78592 509 2
eISBN 978 1 78450 894 4

Printed and bound in Great Britain

To Deborah Selden Burton (1955–1995)

My first friend

To all my clients and students

Contents

Foreword by Phil Jones 9

Acknowledgments 15

Author's Note 16

PART I: FRAMEWORK

1. Introduction 19
2. Creative Arts Therapies, Creative Projection, and Aesthetic Distance 29
3. Creative DNA and Perception Differences 35
4. Stages of Creative Process 46
5. Therapeutic Frame 57
6. Elements in Myths, Fairy Tales, and Traditional Stories . . 78
7. How to Go Through the Steps 96

PART II: STEPS OF THE PROCESS

8. Encounter 105
9. Chaos and Order 114
10. Finding and Telling the Story 121
11. Making a Mask 130

12. Placing and Embodying the Mask 138
13. Finding the Moment 147
14. Soundscape 151
15. Environment 158
16. Directing Someone Else 167
17. Obstacle and Helper 175
18. The Edge 184
19. Final Presentation/Ritual 194
20. Afterwards 202

PART III: ALUMNI WRITINGS

PART IV: ADDITIONAL RESOURCES

References 237
Subject Index 245
Author Index 249

Foreword

This book invites the reader to participate in a rich, active combining of thought, personal reflection, creative endeavor, professional growth, and development. My approach to creating a foreword reflects these different experiences of "The Story Within."

Reading it reminded me that stories and myths are not inherently benign. We all have had the experience of being told stories that form a strong element of powerful groups' maintenance of narratives that oppress and "other" those who are different from themselves. As this book notes, fairy stories and ancient myths have "many limitations and blind spots in terms of gender, race, culture, sexual orientation, and identity" (p.81). An acknowledgment of the deep potency of story is visible in the ways dominant cultures use every means they can to control it through censorship, ownership of the media, or by creating traditions which demarcate who can hold the role of storyteller. Dramatist and systems change worker Saltmarshe takes a view of stories that challenges, and is markedly different from this: it is one which resonates with "The Story Within." She argues that we no longer live in a world of "passively inherited stories" and that "we're increasingly creating and sharing our own on a daily basis" (2018, p.10). She positions story and myth as a means of engendering positive change. They can enable marginalized experiences and voices to take on forms that are meaningful for the story makers themselves and which communicate effectively to others: "story has many different qualities…it's a direct route to our emotions, and therefore important to decision-making. It creates meaning out of patterns. It coheres communities. It engenders empathy across difference. It enables the possible to feel probable in ways our rational minds can't comprehend" (2018, p.4). This book is a testament to such potencies: how particular routes into story and myth can create change through the engendering of powerful meanings, emotions, and relationships.

One of the many strengths of the different chapters is that they are deeply participatory, and as I read them, I found myself following the many opportunities offered to reflect and to create. In Chapter 8, for example, we are invited to prepare for the next step of the journey:

> Before we begin the *Story Within* process it is important to get a sense of our relationship to our own creativity. To do this, here are the steps to follow (you can do this alone or with your circle of support):
>
> 1. Write down three words that come to mind quickly when you think of creativity (allow no more than one to two minutes for this).
>
> 2. How close to your body do you feel your creativity is right now (far away in another room, inside your belly, on the tips of your fingers…)? Indicate this physically.
>
> 3. Where in your body do you feel your creativity (hands, breath, head)? (p.107)

Reading the book is often akin to being in the presence of an experienced and knowledgeable mentor and companion. It is challenging and warm, offering dialogue and thoughtful accompaniment to the many discoveries it shares and enables. I was very taken, for example, by the book's invitations to explore "the Edge." In Chapter 18, the concept is described as having different meanings:

> It can be the outside limit of an object, area, or surface, the border, or the sharpened side of a blade or weapon. As a verb it implies moving gradually, carefully, to advance slowly. All these meanings are applicable for the way the "Edge" is used in the *Story Within* process. When we face a hidden and potentially traumatic part of ourselves, we need to approach it gradually and over time so that we feel safe and prepared. (p.186)

Silverman invites reflection as she asks the reader to consider their own stories and process, in this instance: "As therapists it is important to recognize where our own personal Edge is. We cannot go anywhere with those we work with unless we have explored these areas within ourselves" (p.191). Though I no longer work as a therapist, I found myself reflecting on this. In Chapter 1 Silverman says that "Everyone has a story" (p.20). So here is one of mine, offered as an illustration of how reading this book is a many-faceted experience.

Though I have never directly smoked a cigarette, I have always found the smell reassuring. I am told that I was born into a room filled with the smoke of relatives' cigarettes anxiously keeping my mother company after the loss of two previous children, both girls: though I think my connection is probably not from that far back. My unconscious association is more probably to do with cigarette smoke, storytelling, and story making. As a child I was terrified of the dark and, willful and agentic, insisted that my parents sat with me and told me stories till I fell asleep. When a story ended, I would know whether they were staying with me for another tale, or they were trying to make an escape, by my monitoring the red light of their cigarette traveling through the dark to my bedroom door. At the time little was known in my community of the dangers of active or passive smoking, so I am not including this small story to accuse my parents of endangerment! I include this sample of my childhood for another reason. When I reflect back on it, I see within it a number of elements that connect with why I found this book riveting and why I think it deeply important.

Because the room was dark, my parents had to draw on their own reservoir of story and could not rely on the content, language, and rhythm of reading aloud from a book. My mother called on a vocabulary of castles and princesses, told to her in childhood, and created, for me, a set of stories of her own made from the woods and animals in the tales she knew. My father's stories were around one format and there were three variations. It was about three men walking along a road, when they vanished to appear in either a desert, a forest, or a strange city. It was the stories embellished and re-imagined out of the traditional narratives' people, places, and journeys that I preferred and demanded. Night after night, over many years, my falling asleep was accompanied by a very small repertoire of the same, repeated stories, delivered by parents whose experience of this process I only accessed many years later, when, whilst engaged in my own therapy, I asked for their side of the story making.

The *Story Within*'s goal is to explore how myths, fairy tales, and traditional stories can "uncover and work with hidden and inaccessible aspects of ourselves" (pp.22–23). When I reflected, stimulated by Chapter 18, my recollection contained many layers and dimensions that connect with my reading of this book. The place of story, for example, connects to how such narratives are passed from one person to another—my mother and father were naturally taking me into their imaginary and cultural worlds. The story making by them was active—they were creating and assembling their stories from a generations-long vocabulary given to them. However, the story making and telling was not general or impersonally traditional: it was also deeply alive within a very specific context. The process was as much about relationship as content: the act of being together, of the story as part of care or reassurance, of presence, and of our parent–child dynamics. In addition, the story experience for me was one where it naturally segued into dream: my parents, the story, the relationship between us formed a safe, liminal state where my fear of the dark, or my fear of falling into a state where I was no longer conscious, was reassured. My childhood dreams often reflected and created dialogue with the stories' images and journeys. Years later, as a client in a drama therapy group, I spontaneously created a story and an image emerged: of myself on the side of a wide expanse of dark water, with two female figures on the far shore, arms stretched out to me. I experienced anxiety and distress, completely unexpected, when enacting the story in the role of myself. I thought about this moment of being a client in a group when reading Silverman's advice that, "if I as the therapist or professor assign a specific interpretation for a symbol that emerges organically from someone else, I am limiting the possibilities and taking away from the person's own discovery. A dark figure or a horse in a dream can have so many different meanings depending on culture and context" (pp.23–24). This is an example of how well the different chapters offer clear and essential guidance for those working therapeutically with story and myth. Her encapsulated wisdom here makes clear the ways meaning is complex, moving over time, and how important it is for the therapist to try not to locate it or pin it down. Multiple associations and meanings emerged for me from this moment of a re-enactment, but some connected straight back to the stories with my parents of decades before. The emergence of the story in a therapy group was within a safe space, relationship, and creative context. Thinking about it whilst reading Silverman's writing enabled, for me, another set of insights into the nature of story. In reflection within the therapy, dialogue between the story that had emerged in the therapy room and my childhood bedtime helped me see and feel the fear of the dark, my sisters who had died before me: how for myself, and, perhaps, unconsciously for my parents, that the anxious, liminal state between consciousness and unconsciousness was helped by the process of story making between us. The enacted story also held for me the previously unacknowledged and unspoken which, through the embodied image, started to become eloquent. It was this story and startling image that initiated a longer exploration of my childhood in therapy, but also resulted in my deciding to start to talk to my parents about their/our silenced experience of loss. My recollection of my childhood and experience of therapy, stimulated by this book, helped me understand how the experiencing of a story within a therapeutic context created a bridge between the enactment world and life outside the therapy space. It was illuminated for me by Silverman's invitation to feel and to reflect, contained in her writing.

The example I've given is a demonstration of how this book offers the reader a wonderful opportunity of involvement and learning. It contains careful insights into processes that develop the theoretical and deep structural insight necessary for a therapist to be a professional, rather than a technician who delivers activities. When chapters explore application, they do so by enabling the reader to be inspired to think through the interactions between personal experience, theory, creativity, and application: insight from Silverman's own depth and range of experience and the accounts of those she has worked with. Chapter 3 includes, for example, a finely articulated framework for us to discover our "creative DNA," divided into categories such as "Perceptions," "Focal lens," and "Time factor." Chapter 4 offers a lucid exploration of the stages of creative processes of the *Story Within*: Preparation; Immersion; Incubation; Illumination; and Verification. These frameworks and explorations enable a sharing of Silverman's expertise and experience, but they also form a journey to assist each reader to develop their own personal and professional insights concerning application. The myriad creative opportunities and invitations to think, design, and work cover a wide-ranging diversity: from mask to embodiment, from play to image making. The chapters open up vistas of experiential working with concepts and practices such as "art-to-art response." The book talks about the importance of creating a "circle of support" of others to guide and help in planning and implementing this area of work, and this book gave me a real sense that its content, and the presence of Silverman within its words, formed a part of my "circle of support."

Saltmarshe articulates a much-needed momentum, involving growing numbers of people having the "means to be storytellers as well as story-listeners…we should seek to enable others to use story to illuminate the lay of their land, to cohere communities, and to re-author the nest of narratives they live in" (2018, p.14). This book is an empowering and lucid part of such a cultural move. It is an inspiring call and guide to action.

Professor Phil Jones
Head of Research Ethics and Governance
University College London, Institute of Education

Reference

Saltmarshe, E. (2018). *Telling the difference: Using story to change systems.* London, UK: Calouste Gulbenkian Foundation.

Acknowledgments

My heartfelt thanks to all my clients and students who taught me how to listen, learn, make mistakes, and repair. To Jane Evans, my wonderful editor at Jessica Kingsley Publishers, who reached out to me across the continent to see if I had a book in me. Without her initial invitation and continued support throughout the process I would never have written a word. And heartfelt thanks to Emma Scriver, Editorial Assistant and Emma Holak, Senior Production Editor, and all the amazing folks at Jessica Kingsley Publisher. To my first reader, Miriam Hoffer, thank you for your clarity, wisdom, and care; your feedback and suggestions made this a much better book. To my dearest friends, Judy Stone and Marilyn Bronstein, thank you for agreeing to dive into the dark waters of my myth and embody my story with such depth and generosity. To all the other Cronettes, Victoria Block, Joanne Gormley, Karen Knei-Cahana, Vera Kisfalvi, and Ruth Schwarcz, thank you for witnessing me with such love and grace. To my dear friend, Terry Bohbot, who always brings me back to earth, and to Sherry Diamond, my California sister, who has always had my back. To my Spirit Girls, Henny Feldman, Sonia Zylberberg, Diana Yaros, Louise Houle, and others, our singing and praying always lifts me up. To all my colleagues at the Department of Creative Arts Therapies at Concordia University, it has been a pleasure to know you and work together. To my parents, Arthur and Rita Silverman, who instilled a love of the arts and inspire me every day with their integrity and enthusiasm for life. To my brother Jonathan who has always been there for me even when I was not with myself, and his amazing family. To my son Joshua, his wife Vicky, and my daughter Rebecca, you are my heart. And finally, to my husband, John, who is my rock and has kept me honest and laughing for all these years.

Author's Note

In addition to this book I have also created a documentary film about the *Story Within* process. While certainly not essential, it might be useful to watch the film while you are reading the book as a way of seeing the process in action. The film follows six people as they immerse themselves as characters in self-selected and personally meaningful myths or fairytales. Although it does not go through all of the steps outlined in the book, you can witness many of the creative exercises and watch as individuals embark on a very personal journey of self-discovery. You can also see how the group supports each other and how they use art-to-art responses. The film and book are meant to complement each other and be helpful as you enter your own *Story Within* adventure.

The Story Within—Myth and Fairy Tale in Therapy © 2004

Produced, written, and directed by Yehudit Silverman (53 minutes)

Original music composed by Yehudit Silverman, Jeffery May, and John Rundell

Cinematographer: Martin Duckworth

Sound: Glenn Hodgins

Editor: Andre Elias

English with French subtitles

[Add info about downloading from JKP if this goes ahead]

Part I

FRAMEWORK

CHAPTER 1

Introduction

I was alone on a sailboat 70 miles from land. The waves were over 15 ft and the mast had just broken. What was left of the sailboat was just a shell. I held on as the waves tossed me back and forth and looked out on an endless sea. Radio communication was broken, the motor just 6-horse power, I was helpless. At 23 I had felt invincible but, in this moment, I knew I could die. I screamed out for help, I prayed, and at one point I found myself chanting in a language I did not speak. It was as if in that moment I became someone else, someone ancient and powerful who was coming through me. In the distance I heard a powerboat and I was saved...

Finding Meaning

The above story is true and was a pivotal moment that forced me to reckon with a sense of meaning and purpose to my life. Why was I here? Was there a quest, a search, a path that I needed to discover? And how could I find this? And who or what powerful force came through me in my moment of terror? It was as if I was me but also someone else at the same time, some archetypal mythic character that was summoned by my predicament. As a dancer, an adventurer, and someone who felt lost within myself, I had no answers, no guiding mentor to lead me to my path. And despite not feeling I was on a path, when I was faced with death on the ocean something propelled me forward, giving me the courage and ruthless belief that there was a path for me to follow, and a quest to discover. All of us face these moments of truth when the day-to-day tasks slip away, and we are forced to take stock of who we are and where our life is leading us.

It could be the sudden death of a loved one, an illness, a breakup, a religious experience, or disillusionment with a belief system. In these pivotal moments there is an opening to a mythic sense of being. Questions of meaning and purpose become important and we realize that perhaps we are on a quest, that there is a path that feels true to who we are, and that if we are not on this path, we feel lost. Myths, fairy tales, and ancient stories from around the world speak of a quest: a journey fraught with obstacles, demons, and monsters. As Campbell (2008, 2011, 2017) and others have brought into public consciousness, these ancient stories are still relevant today and can be an essential guide for our current struggles and challenges.

Stories

Everyone has a story. We all live by narratives that define who we are and how we approach the world. Our reactions to what we encounter come out of these narratives. And yet, our emotional reactions often surprise and challenge us because they seem to come out of nowhere. In my work as a therapist I discovered that there are underlying and often hidden stories that remain inaccessible. It is these hidden stories that truly control how we approach and interact with the world. Within these hidden stories are the traumas, emotional wounds, and difficult memories and experiences that we have blocked off from our consciousness. We cannot see or feel them, yet they hold us firmly in their grip, leading us to react as if we are fighting for our very survival. While talk therapy and addressing personal issues in a direct manner may be helpful, working only cognitively can keep us from making a true visceral connection to that which lies buried and out of reach. How do we access what remains unconscious and hidden? How can we find a safe way to approach our deepest fears? For much of our human history our fears have been expressed in our myths, fairy tales, and traditional stories. From Persephone to the Ugly Duckling, the themes and challenges within these stories resonated with our own life. In more recent times, knowledge of the human mind and psyche has grown, and the ideas of modern psychology imbue nearly every aspect of society. Therapeutic models and ideals abound, and while the growing acceptance of the field is encouraging, in its rise, something may have been forgotten. In the pursuit of scientific acceptance, the primal and fundamental nature of the narrative and story has been left by the wayside. Or the stories have been censored and stripped of their dark and more sinister elements. The fairy tales reimagined by Disney left out the most important aspects: the monsters, demons, ambiguous endings, and immoral characters, all of which allowed us to truly explore the chaotic and challenging aspects of our existence. It is these darker elements of the stories that allow us to explore these darker elements within ourselves (Silverman, 2006).

The power of myth, fairy tales, and traditional stories is that they give form to archaic, atavistic fears, anxieties, and longings. Often these are too frightening to confront directly but we can identify with the protagonist in the story as they face demons and obstacles on their journey. By entering a fictional world that contains timeless and essential themes we connect with something larger than ourselves. This connection with something larger allows us to work with both the conscious and the unconscious at the same time. The symbols and metaphors become interwoven with the real-life situation, and the profound intersects with the prosaic (Bettelheim, 1976/2010; Conrad, 2017; Marks, 2017). The notion of a collective unconscious of universal patterns and symbols was an integral aspect of Jung's (1953/2014) work as a psychoanalyst. With his patients he explored how these elemental psychic themes manifest in behavior or interaction with the outside world. One of Jung's archetypal forms that is relevant when working with stories is the idea of the "shadow" (Bollas, 2017; Dunne, 2015). This dark, unknown, and potentially troubling part of our psyche is often denied and projected onto others. A major goal in Jungian analysis is to reintegrate the shadow and, when this is done effectively, we can become "whole" by bringing together parts of ourselves that were split or disconnected (Casement, 2012; David, 2017; Donati, 2004). This notion of integrating the shadow or that which was hidden and inaccessible is an integral part of the *Story Within* process.

One key element of most myths, fairy tales, and traditional stories is the idea of a quest or journey. The protagonist must go through a series of challenges, and obstacles. What often initiates this transformational journey is the poignant, and often disturbing, moment when humans and the supernatural meet. Usually this is not an easy interaction, the familiar is challenged and disrupted. It is this disruption of the "norm" that allows for the protagonist to change. This is similar to the psychoanalytic notion that it is necessary for someone to go through a process of disintegration or falling apart before they can be reintegrated and healed (Caldwell, 2018; Green, 2018; Meredith-Owen, 2011; Winnicott, 2016). And wisely, the narratives in myths, fairy tales, and traditional stories often move back and forth between a disruption of the familiar order into a time of disintegration and chaos, then back to a new type of integration or order. This movement between chaos and order, conscious and unconscious, profound and prosaic, is what makes these stories archetypal and timeless (Baciu, 2017). In many indigenous cultures traditional stories were passed on from generation to generation through oral storytelling, expressing cultural beliefs, values, customs, rituals, and history (Corntassel, 2009). There are many diverse aboriginal and indigenous groups across the world, and each have a unique culture with specific stories that relate to their spiritual world view. In some shamanic traditions, specific stories are told in a ritual manner to facilitate healing, both mental and physical (Dhungana and Yamphu, 2016). Similarly, for Estés (2008, 2010), a Jungian analyst, folklorist, and author, stories and storytelling are essential for health and wellbeing. So perhaps, as the Nigerian novelist and poet Ben Okri (1996) offers, "without stories we would go mad…"

The *Story Within* Approach

> Somewhere hidden in the depths of each story lies a treasure waiting to be discovered.

This book is an introduction to an arts-based therapeutic approach called the *Story Within*. The goal is to use myths, fairy tales, and traditional stories to uncover and work with hidden and inaccessible aspects of ourselves. I began developing this approach as a creative arts therapist working in hospital settings and in private practice with children, adolescents, and adults dealing with diverse psychological and physical issues. Most recently I have expanded to working with communities around the issue of suicide, interfaith and cross-cultural dialogue, and intergenerational trauma. For the last 20 years as part of my position as a professor in the Creative Arts Therapies Department at Concordia University in Montreal, I taught a class in this approach to graduate students. In addition, I am grateful to have been invited to offer workshops internationally.

> However, in truth the process began way before then when I was lost at sea and some strange presence came through me… Perhaps that was a beginning and the process evolved by itself, growing inside of me as I moved through my life… What I do know is that it never started as a concept, a theory, an idea, but rather found its way organically as a way to reach others and at the same time to reach inside myself…

As I have confessed, this approach never started out as a concept and yet here I am now dissecting and cutting up what emerged organically into designated parts and segments. I realize this is necessary and, I hope, helpful to frame what will be a direct experiential entry into the process. Unlike many other therapeutic frameworks, this approach integrates all the arts so that personal learning and meaning making comes through the senses and the perceptions rather than just cognitively. Using all the creative mediums allows for a different type of knowledge to emerge, one that is visceral and long lasting. The focus is on creative process and creative uncertainty as a means for transformation. Therefore, it is essential that the process of discovery not be limited by one perspective or interpretation. And while Jungian archetypes, the shadow, and individuation are crucial building blocks, the *Story Within* does not adhere to any one psychological theory or interpretation. In my work I found that if I as the therapist or professor assign a specific interpretation for a symbol that emerges organically from someone else, I am limiting the possibilities and taking away from the person's own discovery. A dark figure or a horse in a dream can have so many different meanings depending on culture and context. How can we possibly know what it truly means for someone else? For the *Story Within* approach the focus is on learning our own "creative DNA" (Tharp, 2003) and discovering our own symbolic language and meanings. Many therapists choose the story or stories for their clients to work with. However, in the *Story Within* it is the client who chooses the story. The process of finding the "right story" is an integral part of the therapy. Each client works on their own personal story instead of working as a part of a group on a collective story.

The *Story Within* process involves an in-depth relationship with a self-selected myth, fairy tale, or traditional story that evokes a personal sense of relevance, although not understood. The identification of the story, the character in it, and the dramatic moment that is felt to be the most significant, all involve a personal quest similar to the heroic mythic journey described by Campbell (2008, 2011), Leeming (2005, 2010, 2014), Gilligan and Dilts (2009), and Hartman and Zimberoff (2009). These authors suggest that the classic mythic journeys all involve an intense search in which the hero (meant here to be non-gender-specific) discovers something important about themselves. Similarly, those of us who embark on the *Story Within* method choose our own stories and become heroes in our own personal mythic quest. The process entails a deep relationship with a carefully chosen character as a way of working with unconscious personal material. Without being required to understand or make the character/life connection, we enjoy creating masks, art work, costumes, dramatic scenes, sculpts (a gestural pose or stance that is either still or moving and can include a sound or word), music, and movement as we identify with our character. This "not knowing" and trust in the journey itself allows the depth work to be done and allows the internal story, the one that is hidden, buried, and hardest to access, to be gradually revealed, often for the first time.

The *Story Within* approach provides safety and distance, so we can immerse ourselves in the creative process, and not have the anxiety of directly facing our personal problem. In the process of creatively and emotionally engaging with our character's problem and challenges, we see things from the character's point of view. As we live the reality of our character's journey, we find ourselves confronting our character's trauma or deepest fear which we gradually realize is our own. Approaching therapy as an inquiry, a journey into the unknown, with the therapist as a guide and a witness, provides the autonomy and courage to face inner demons. May (1980/1994) believed that insight breeds anxiety and guilt due to the inherent struggle between what we consciously hold on to and some new thought, or belief, wanting to be born. Despite the joy of the actual insight, there is anxiety about letting go of old patterns of behavior, even destructive ones. The gradual emerging of insight in the *Story Within* approach gives room for that initial anxiety and struggle so that insights can be slowly integrated into perceptions and actions.

About This Book

> The only true way to learn about the *Story Within* approach is to go through the process…

After many years of working with the *Story Within* approach in many different settings, I decided it was time to try and solidify the specific theory and practice in a book format. It is meant to be a practical resource and guide for clinicians, therapists, creative arts therapists, and community workers. I have designed the book to be both a step-by-step guide to the process that you, the reader, can follow at your own pace, and also a more didactic framework for you to understand the theory and practical application. The only true way to learn about the *Story Within* approach is to go through the process. Without experiencing it, there is no way to understand how each step feels and the impact of working profoundly with a chosen character. To be able to guide others using aspects of this process, you as the therapist, clinician, or community worker need to experience first-hand what it is like to uncover your own hidden story. This takes courage and a willingness to explore your own creativity and unconscious material. To help others we must be as aware as possible of our own stories and narratives, so we don't impose them on our clients. We all have blind spots, parts of ourselves that we cannot see, that always remain just out of sight yet haunt us throughout our lives. The *Story Within* process can help to reveal these blind spots and perhaps make us better and more effective at helping others. The steps of the process are designed to provide a safe and gradual structure for deep personal exploration. Therefore, it is essential to be in a secure and stable state of mind before embarking on any of the exercises. The best way to go through the steps is with a small support group of other health and community workers. You can support each other, be witness for each other's creativity, and share feelings and insights as they emerge (more about how to set this up in Chapter 5, "Therapeutic Frame," and Chapter 7, "How to Go Through the Steps"). And if you feel that you are in a fragile state, then please find a therapist or professional who can provide support.

I have divided the book into four main parts: (I) Framework; (II) Steps of the Process; (III) Alumni Writings; and (IV) Additional Resources. I would suggest you start from the beginning since the framework covers all the underlying concepts that inform the process. Without an understanding of these concepts and the terminology, it will be much harder to go through the steps. And the sequence of the steps is important and is intentionally designed to take you from one stage to the next in a safe and gradual manner. It may be helpful to view the video, *The Story Within—Myth and Fairy Tale in Therapy* (Silverman, 2004a), and read its related publication (Silverman, 2004b), as a companion to the book. The video follows six people as they go through the process and it can be useful to see examples of the process in action. The book can also be an integral part of the training to be a certified practitioner of the *Story Within* method.

Creativity

"Odd how the creative power at once brings the whole universe to order."

Virginia Woolf (1882–1941)

Everyone is creative. There is an innate calling to respond to the world through some sort of creative medium. Sadly, this creative impulse is often stifled, or worse, actively discouraged, in childhood by teachers, parents, and society in the goal of producing "successful" or "goal oriented" children. However, the natural creative play of children cannot totally be repressed or forgotten and comes alive when we spontaneously make sandcastles by the sea, dance in our room where no one can see us, or doodle in long meetings. The creative imagination is within our DNA, but it needs to be nurtured and encouraged (Tharp, 2003). Creative arts therapies is a field that recognizes the inherent value of the arts as necessary for health and wellbeing. As creative arts therapists we are trained to work in clinical and community settings using the arts as a therapeutic tool (see more about creative arts therapies training in the "Additional Resources" section). As a registered dance and drama therapist, and as an artist working with documentary film, mask making, dance, and music, I have seen the power of the arts to transform individuals and communities. As someone who has always worked with stories, I have seen that combining the power of the creative process with the potent and ancient content of myth and fairy tale has proven an effective way to access and work with the hidden stories that often unconsciously control our lives.

You may be someone who already has a creative practice, or you may feel that creativity is reserved for others who are "talented" or "artists." Sadly, this belief can keep you from discovering your own natural creative voice and the joy that comes from using your expressive muscles. The *Story Within* is an arts-based approach and is appropriate and beneficial to anyone even if you have not explored any creative mediums since childhood. The structure of the process provides an opportunity to rediscover your creativity, explore diverse mediums, and express inner feelings through non-verbal avenues. It does not require an expertise or even familiarity with any or all mediums. All that is necessary is a willingness to connect with an inherent part of yourself that wants to explore, to discover, to be open, and to play.

To reach across the page, I have decided to include aspects of my clinical work with a diverse range of clients. For each step and exercise, I begin with a brief clinical vignette of how this aspect of the process was used in my clinical work (with no breach of client confidentiality). And along with you, the reader, I will also go through the steps and stages of the *Story Within* and will include very brief excerpts from my personal process throughout the book. Words on a page are not the same thing as meeting face to face, and although I will not be physically present with you, perhaps sharing some of my own, more personal writings can make us more connected.

> To create, to enter the *Story Within* process, all of us must be willing to fully commit ourselves to the unknown. We don't know where we are going or where we will end up. All we know is that there is a path and there are those who have gone before, fought similar demons, and found hidden treasures. Somewhere hidden in the depths of each story lies a treasure waiting to be discovered. There is not one treasure but many, a different treasure for each of us who dares to dig deep enough. I wish you a wonderful, transformative adventure…

CHAPTER 2

Creative Arts Therapies, Creative Projection, and Aesthetic Distance

He sat in the waiting room, shoulders hunched, holding tightly on to his mother's hand. He didn't want to leave her when I came to get him, and she had to promise that she would stay right there until he was finished with our therapy session. Reluctantly, this six-year-old boy walked beside me trailing his hand along the wall. I asked him about stories and he immediately launched into an intricate tale about Superman. As he told me the story, he began to leap around the hallway pretending his coat was Superman's cape. For the next few weeks we worked with this character who was sent from a dying alien planet to Earth where he is adopted and gradually realizes he has secret powers. This young boy's parents had recently told him that he was adopted, and he was confused and worried that they might give him up. He identified with Superman coming from an alien planet and not knowing fully who he was. In one session he created a shield and cape for Superman made from red and blue fabric with glitter and photos of himself as a baby and images of Superman. When he put on the cape and shield, he went over to the window and looked out and asked in a soft voice, "Where am I from? Where is my planet? Who are my real parents?" Then he stopped, his lips trembled and his eyes watered, but then he touched his shield with his hands and told me, "But I do have secret powers and I can help the world." The character of Superman helped him to express the complexity of his feelings about learning he was adopted and also to make peace with it by connecting with his own inner strength.

Creative Projection

"The aim of art is to represent not the outward appearance of things, but their inward significance."

Aristotle, Greek philosopher (384–322 BC)

One of the basic elements of creative arts therapies is the idea of "creative projection." Jones (2007; 2016), Malchiodi (2011), and others describe this as a process in which we project aspects of ourselves or our experience onto a creative medium. By doing this we externalize our inner world onto a creative form that we can work with, whether it be a dramatic role, an art piece, or a musical composition. Working creatively, we are active, engaging all our senses, and through each medium exploring and expressing our inner world. In creative arts therapies the goal is to foster the development of a profound relationship between our inner emotional world and our external creative form. This allows us both a high degree of safety when working through difficult material, and the ability to discover new perspectives about our situation or problem. Thus, in creative arts therapies "creative projection" is an essential therapeutic tool and provides the primary medium through which change occurs. It offers an opportunity to project hidden and often shameful feelings onto a creative form without having to verbally articulate them. For example, a mother I worked with whose children needed to be in foster care created collages and movements that expressed both her grief at losing her children and her shame at not being able to take care of them. Having a creative form outside of herself that was at the same time deeply connected to her feelings became a kind of "transitional object," imbued with a subjective personal significance that includes both "me" and "not me" (Winnicott, 2016). The projection of difficult feelings onto an unthreatening object or role is a safe way to gain perspective and its symbolic expression becomes a powerful means of communication. In contrast, traditional psychology views projection very differently. It is often seen as a defense mechanism, a way for clients to deny their own feelings by putting them outside onto someone else. In fact, the goal of many psychotherapeutic approaches is to help clients gain insight about their projections and to reclaim disowned feelings or parts of themselves through discussion or analysis. Yalom (2005) and others describe projection as an unconscious process that consists of projecting some of our own inner conflicts, and unresolved feelings, onto someone else without recognizing that we are doing this. Therefore, the use of projection in traditional psychology and the use of creative projection in creative arts therapies is quite different. However, the ultimate goal is the same in terms of working to provide an opportunity for change and healing.

> "If you bring forth what is within you, what you bring forth will save you. If you don't bring forth what is within you, what you don't bring forth will destroy you."
>
> The Gospel of St Thomas

Creative projection can be particularly helpful when working with trauma. Survivors of trauma or abuse are often conflicted between wanting to return to the pre-traumatic world before the trauma or abuse, and an unconscious tendency to re-experience the abuse through nightmares or destructive relationships (Enns, 2018; Jennings, 2018). This inner conflict plays out as a need to avoid pain, and yet at the same time, a need to resolve the painful experience. For example, an adolescent I worked with, who had been abused as a child, made a doll to represent Sleeping Beauty. In some sessions she would lovingly lie the doll down in a soft bed to sleep and in other sessions she would throw the doll against the wall and tell her to "wake up!" Through the creative projection of the doll she was ultimately able to work through her desire to "sleep" and dissociate from what happened to her and to "wake up" and face it so she could move on. She was able to project these contrasting feelings onto one object. An artistic creation, unlike language, has the capacity to contain paradox, complexity, and opposing points of view in one form (Chamberlain *et al.*, 2018; McNiff, 2012; 2017). The variety of creative mediums offered can open the door to many clients who would never engage in more traditional verbal therapies. Those who have suffered trauma or abuse may be so wounded by their previous trauma they believe the world is unsafe, people are dangerous, no one can or will help them, and it is inevitable that they will be attacked again (Knight, 2018). Rather than continuing to disassociate from their traumatic memories, through creative projection they can learn to express experiences which are beyond words. They can break the taboo of secrecy through drama, art, music, and dance, in a safe and controlled way, and can acknowledge and re-examine their trauma so that they become empowered and can move on in their lives.

Creative projection can be an immediate spontaneous expression or a cumulative process that is developed over time. The *Story Within* approach is a sustained and longer-term creative projection. Once we have chosen the story, character, and moment, we stay with it for several weeks or months depending on the need and circumstances. Having a sustained projection allows us to potentially access more hidden and inaccessible parts of ourselves. If we have experienced trauma or patterns of behavior that are destructive but tenacious, this approach can help to access buried feelings in a safe and gradual way. Often there are layers in our psyche, and it takes time to sift through each layer to get to the underlying narrative. Working with a fictional, mythic character and through diverse creative mediums allows us to determine the timing and rhythm of our own process. We identify with and develop a deep relationship with a single character. This makes the personal projection onto the character particularly intense and creates a setting in which we can connect with uncomfortable feelings without being threatened. There is also reassurance: here is a character who feels the same way we do.

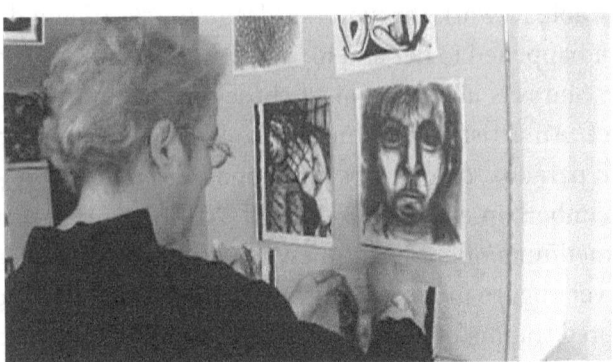

Gale Ostroff with artwork

Aesthetic Distance

> Creative projection offers a unique opportunity to simultaneously establish a strong emotional engagement and a safe emotional distance.

Drama therapist Robert Landy (1996, 2010, 2017) proposes that finding a balance, or aesthetic distance between being "under-distanced" (being overwhelmed by emotions) and "over-distanced" (little access to emotions or feelings), is essential for healing. One of the ways of developing aesthetic distance is working with creative projection. In a creative arts therapies session, once the medium is chosen and the creative projection is underway, the therapist monitors how clients engage emotionally with their personal material (Henson and Fitzpatrick, 2016). Creative projection offers a unique opportunity to simultaneously establish a strong emotional engagement and a safe emotional distance. For example, if someone needs more emotional engagement, they can enter deeply into a role as an actor, use their body in movement, or sing an original song. In contrast, if they need more distance, they can be the director, or witness, or make a drawing, or listen to recorded music. The creative possibilities are endless and allow the therapist and client to shift easily between the cognitive and the emotional. One session might intensify the emotional engagement while another might encourage emotional distance. This is especially important when working with trauma. Reliving trauma can lead to a flood of anxiety, and instead of integrating the experience, the client will just be re-traumatized. Avoidance does not work either, as the client will be unable to deal with other life traumas. Creative arts therapies and creative projection offer a middle ground, addressing trauma without the accompanying overwhelming anxiety. Since clients have a sense of control through manipulation of symbolic materials and creative mediums, they can prevent emotional flooding or re-traumatization. Through the techniques of creative projection, clients maintain a balance between emotional engagement and distance to be able to access, and eventually integrate, disassociated parts of themselves (Ali *et al.*, 2018; Bailey, 2007; Frydman and Mayor, 2017). In my work as a creative arts therapist, I found that using myth, fairy tale, and traditional stories provided the right amount of aesthetic distance so that whatever emotions, memories, or sensations arose, they were not overwhelming. Gradually, and over time, the story that was hidden, shameful, and buried was revealed and could be seen and worked with in a safe and transformative way.

> As I write these words, I struggle to find a way to maintain aesthetic distance. I want to convey the concepts, but I also want to make it personal, relevant, and accessible. Can my words be both? Do I have to choose a stance, one lens to see through? I have always felt more at home in the transition between water, land, and air. If only I could swim, run, and fly the ideas so that they magically find you, the reader, in whatever place we can meet…

CHAPTER 3

Creative DNA and Perception Differences

When I entered the small, dim hospital room, I saw him down on his knees rocking back and forth and moaning. A beautiful boy of six with curly dark hair, I wasn't sure if he knew I was present. He made no eye contact, did not turn in my direction, just continued his rocking and quiet moaning. I was a relatively new therapist, and this was one of my first individual patients, so I was eager to connect. However, when I moved closer to him, he let out a piercing scream and I retreated. I realized I had to find a way to engage without making eye contact, without getting closer, and since he was non-verbal, without words. I tried echoing his moans, but this just made him more agitated and he rocked faster. Finally, I decided to start a rhythm with my feet on the ground. He continued to rock and moan but very gradually his rocking matched the rhythm of my feet. We continued with this rhythmic connection for the rest of the session and in our future work together. It was this rhythmic connection that allowed us to gradually move physically closer and have more extensive periods of eye contact. Even though his diagnosis of autism left him isolated in his internal world, we were able to find ways of making rhythmic, often playful conversations. His family joined in for some of the sessions and this provided all of them with a new way to communicate. I learned from this young boy that part of my job as a therapist is to discover what perception and mediums truly communicate for my client. I came into the session looking forward to moving and doing art together and yet sound and rhythm were the only avenues that he responded to.

Each Person's Unique Way of Experiencing the World

As we go through life, we each have a unique way of experiencing the world. Although we may not be conscious of it, we each filter our environment and our interactions differently. According to Twyla Tharp (2003), a renowned choreographer, we are all hardwired with specific creative codes that are as solidly imprinted in us as the genetic code that determines our height and eye color. The only difference is that these codes govern our creative impulses and the mediums and forms we choose and the way we use them. So far, her theories cannot be proven; however, I have found her basic concepts helpful as a way of understanding and reflecting on our own creative process. I suspect most of us never get a handle on our creative identity or the particular preferences that inform how we engage with the world. Having self-knowledge about our own unique creative impulses can help us identify the common threads in our own patterns, both positive and self-destructive, and reflect on areas where we are strong and where we are weak. For example, Tharp (2003) herself prefers things to be black and white, to make clear distinctions, and to divide the world into opposites. This preference, she believes, is part of her creative DNA (Tharp, 2003). For others, living in ambiguity, seeing the gray, enjoying not having clear distinctions, is part of their creative DNA. Each one of us is unique with a specific set of patterns, preferences, and innate skills that determine the way we create. Some of us will see the world from a great distance, a large sweeping view, or the big picture, while others will focus intensely on what is right in front of us very close up and detailed. Both points of view are valid and interesting—it just depends on what calls to us and what feels authentic. Perhaps we can think of our creative DNA as essential to our health and wellbeing. Just as we need to ensure nutritional and physical health, we need a way of determining our creative health. The concept of creative DNA and examining our own creative process provides an opportunity to discover what we need to be creative and how each medium affects us. This understanding can lead us to foster our creativity as a way of responding to our experiences in an authentic and healing way.

As a framework for us to discover our creative DNA in the *Story Within* process, I have divided our exploration into the following categories: Perceptions (visual, auditory, tactile, kinesthetic, emotional, smell and taste); Creative DNA (focal lens, time factor, product/process, internal/external, and emergent/structured); Focal lens; Time factor; Product/Process; Internal/External; and Emergent/Structured). There could be many more categories and this list is certainly not complete. However, I have found these categories to be most helpful as a framework for the creative exercises and reflections for the *Story Within*. There is no right or wrong creative DNA. All preferences in all categories are equal. There is no hierarchy or "good" or "bad." It is important to let go of all judgment and expectations and just be open to discovery.

Perceptions

Even though we use all our perceptions as we go through life, we each have innate or acquired preferences, and discovering our preferences can be helpful as a way of understanding ourselves and our relationships. Here is a brief outline of the eight perceptions I have identified as being crucial for the *Story Within*. I invite you to look at each one and see if you can identify your own preferences and perhaps those of your clients and loved ones. I have included a questionnaire at the end of the chapter that may be helpful in identifying your perception preferences.

Visual

You are the ones who notice everything visual in your environment—the colors, the shapes, the person sitting on the corner of the street. For you, "seeing" is essential. It is your primary way of experiencing the world. Whereas you can become aware of the other perceptions, the visual is so natural, so unconscious, that you do not have to think about it. You may use the words "I see what you're saying" or "I see what you mean." You may not be a visual artist but the visual is very satisfying and necessary for you to experience the world.

Auditory

You are the ones who hear everything in your environment—the bird songs, the background music, the sound of voices. For you, "hearing" is essential. It is your primary way of experiencing the world. Whereas you can become aware of the other perceptions, the auditory is so natural, so unconscious, that you do not have to think about it. You may use the words "I hear what you're saying" or "I hear what you mean." You may not be a musician but the auditory is very satisfying and necessary for you to experience the world.

Tactile

You are the ones who touch everything in your environment—you pay attention to the texture of the wood, the feel of the fabric, the smoothness of skin. For you, "touching" is essential. It is your primary way of experiencing the world. Whereas you can become aware of the other perceptions, the tactile is so natural, so unconscious, that you do not have to think about it. You may use the words "I am touched by what you're saying." You may not be a tactile artist but the tactile is very satisfying and necessary for you to experience the world.

Kinesthetic

You are the ones who notice everything in terms of your experience of your own body—the feeling of your muscles as you stretch, the feeling of wind on your skin, the parts of your body that move as you breathe. For you, "sensing your internal body" is essential. It is your primary way of experiencing the world. Whereas you can become aware of the other perceptions, the kinesthetic is so natural, so unconscious, that you do not have to think about it. You may use the words "I feel that in my gut" or "I can't breathe around this person." You may not be a dancer, but the kinesthetic is very satisfying and necessary for you to experience the world.

Emotional

You are the ones who notice everything in terms of emotions—your own and those of others. You feel the pain of someone else's story, you feel your angry response to something you read, you can easily discern between different feelings and label them appropriately and use your emotional information to guide your thinking and behavior. It is your primary way of experiencing the world. Whereas you can become aware of the other perceptions, the emotional is so natural, so unconscious, that you do not have to think about it. You may use the words "I'm really angered by what you're saying" or "I feel really hurt by your words." You may not be a therapist but the emotional is very satisfying and necessary for you to experience the world.

Conceptual

You are the ones who notice everything in terms of a concept. You can easily analyze hypothetical situations or abstract concepts to compile insight. You understand patterns of thought and are excited by ideas and intellectual discussion. For you, "understanding" is essential. It is your primary way of experiencing the world. Whereas you can become aware of the other perceptions, the conceptual is so natural, so unconscious, that you do not have to think about it. You may use the words "I don't understand what you're saying" or "I see the pattern in your story." You may not be an academic but the conceptual is very satisfying and necessary for you to experience the world.

Smell

You are the ones who notice everything in terms of smell. You can easily identify situations and memories according to a corresponding smell. For you, smell is essential. It is your primary way of experiencing the world. Whereas you can become aware of the other perceptions, the sense of smell is so natural, so unconscious, that you do not have to think about it. You may consistently comment on odors and actively smell what is before you. You may not work with smell professionally, but the sense of smell is very satisfying and necessary for you to experience the world.

Taste

You are the ones who notice everything in terms of taste. Food and the corresponding sense of taste for each food is extremely important. You can easily identify distinct types of taste sensations and differentiate specific spices and experience situations and memories according to a corresponding taste. For you, taste is essential. It is your primary way of experiencing the world. Whereas you can become aware of the other perceptions, the sense of taste is so natural, so unconscious, that you do not have to think about it. You may consistently comment on taste and actively taste what is before you. You may not be a professional cook, but the sense of taste is very satisfying and necessary for you to experience the world.

∼

Please don't worry if you have no idea which perception is most dominant. I present this information as a framework that I have found to be helpful in understanding ourselves, our relationships, and in working therapeutically with clients. For example, if you are someone whose primary way of experiencing the world is emotional and your partner is conceptual, you may find that often you have trouble with communication. The actual words and ways of understanding the world are different and therefore it can be difficult to make sense of what your partner is saying. Once you become more aware of your own and your partner's perceptive preferences, then it can be easier to find new pathways to understanding each other.

I suggest you play with this and pay attention over the next week as to what perceptions are most active. You may notice one or two that are most dominant, several that are bit less, and one that is quite underused. For some of you this discovery will be immediate and by the first day of exploration you will know your creative preferences. For others it may remain very vague and not clear. Not to worry—one of the goals of the *Story Within* is to discover your creative DNA through all the creative exercises outlined in the book. Please keep track of how the different mediums affect you and your own personal process of creation. Keeping a journal will help you identify your own creative DNA!

Working with Clients — Perceptions

In terms of working with clients, if you as a therapist are primarily visual you may be inadvertently imposing your preferred perception onto your clients. For example, I had another young boy who was suffering from severe anxiety and in working with him I would look over his drawings, or movements, and ask if he wanted to "see" them. He continually said "no." However, I thought it was "important" that he "look" and "see" what he had done. It was only when I recognized my own visual preference that I understood I was imposing my preference on him! Once that was clear I could let that go and allow his preference (kinesthetic) to emerge which was empowering for him and helped to build alliance and trust.

Creative DNA
Focal Lens
Close Up
You are the ones who notice the details on the tree in front of you, the particular design of the bark or leaves. You prefer to narrow down your focus to one thing at a time and pay attention to the details. You may even bring yourself closer to an object, bend down to see it more clearly, or bring it closer to the eyes. This close-up focus and the details are very satisfying and essential for you to make sense of the world.

Distant Focus
You are the ones who see the whole forest, the way all the trees line up against the sky. You prefer to broaden your focus to include the whole picture. You may even squint, move farther away, or look through a camera so that you get a sweeping view. This distant view of the big picture is satisfying and essential for you to make sense of the world.

Time Factor
Quick/Immediate/Spontaneous
You are the ones whose creative process emerges quickly. You immediately start exploring the mediums and spontaneously put together the form and structure that feels right. You may see it ahead of time or the form may emerge as you work, but the time factor is almost always quick, immediate, and spontaneous. This quick,

immediate, and spontaneous time factor is satisfying and essential for you to make sense of the world.

Slow/Gradual/Thought Out
You are the ones who think before you start creating. You slowly and gradually form an idea and gather materials before you start to work. You may see it ahead of time or the form may emerge as you work, but the time factor is almost always slow, gradual, and thought out. This slow, gradual thought-out time factor is satisfying and essential for you to make sense of the world.

Product/Process
Product as Most Important
You are the ones who have a clear idea of what you want to create, and it is important that you find the right materials, instruments, and movements to bring that idea into the right form. While the process of creating it may be enjoyable and interesting, the most important aspect is the product, the final format and structure. This final product must be exactly how you want it, and achieving that is what is most satisfying and essential for you in making sense of the world.

Process as Most Important
You are the ones who immerse yourself in the process of creating without necessarily a sense of what the product will be. The sensory or cognitive aspect of creating is most important. The sense of discovery, or solving a creative puzzle, is what inspires you. While the final product matters, it is not what engages you the most. The creative process itself is what is most essential and satisfying for you in making sense of the world.

Internal/External
Internally Focussed
You are the ones who must be by yourself to create. You need your own space without external distractions, or interference from others.

This internal focus is necessary for you to be able to concentrate on your own process. External distractions and other people take away your ability to focus. This internal focus is satisfying and essential for you to make sense of the world.

Externally Focussed
You are the ones who love to collaborate with others. You work best in a public space and with others around to give feedback or interact with. Working alone can feel isolating or stifling, and the noise and camaraderie of being with others helps you to focus on your creativity. This external focus is satisfying and essential for you to make sense of the world.

Emergent/Structured
Emergent
You are the ones who have no idea what you will create before you start. You go into the process without a specific structure, format, or design. You trust that the idea, or structure, will emerge as you work. For you, having a specific design or structure ahead of time would be stifling and limiting. You enjoy not knowing what will happen, and this emergent quality is satisfying and essential for you to make sense of the world.

Structured
You are the ones who plan out what you are going to create before you begin. You go into the process with a clear structure, format, and design. You have planned specific steps and know exactly what you are going to do to achieve the final product you want. You trust your plan, your idea, and your ability to make it happen. This structured quality is satisfying and essential for you to make sense of the world.

Working with Clients — Creative DNA
In terms of working with clients, if you as a therapist have a close-up focal preference you may try and impose this on your clients by

asking them to look closely or notice the details. They may need just the opposite: a broader, more distant view so they can perceive the whole picture. Similarly, if you have a quick time factor you may try and rush your client along, becoming impatient with their slower and more gradual way of creating. One of your clients may not care about the final product, while another one cares so much, they spend weeks trying to get it exactly right. In the therapy room your client may need privacy and quiet so they can concentrate, while you may have the urge to keep talking and interacting. Your preference for an external focus can interfere with the necessary internal focus of your client. And lastly, if you are process-oriented and your client is not, you could miss an opportunity to support their inherent need to plan ahead and set up a clear structure. The more we understand our own preferences, the more we can ensure that they do not interfere or get in the way of our clients. And understanding our clients' preferences helps us form a deeper alliance and connection.

Questionnaire for Finding Your Perception Preferences

I developed this questionnaire for my course at Concordia University. Answer whatever you can and don't worry if you have no idea how to answer some of the questions. This is just for your own personal reflection and you can come back to this questionnaire at any time during the *Story Within* process.

For all the questions choose one or two of the aforementioned perceptions: Visual, Auditory, Tactile, Kinesthetic, Emotional, Conceptual, Smell, or Taste. Have fun!

1. What do you feel is your primary way of experiencing the world?

2. Which perception touches you the most and brings up the most emotion (listening to music, seeing a painting, touching something, a beautiful idea or concept, tasting an array of spices, smelling lilacs, seeing someone cry in film, dancing)?

3. Which perception is the most stimulating, gives you energy?

4. Which perception is the most exhausting?

5. Which perception is the most recuperative?

6. Which perception is necessary for something to make sense? (Do you need to see it, read it out loud, feel it with your hands, feel it emotionally, understand the concept, experience it in your body, taste it, smell it?)

7. Which perception is the most foreign—which do you use the least?

8. Which perception are you most expressive with?

9. Which perception is essential in your creative process?

10. Which perception would you like to use more?

I never knew my perception preference was visual. After all, I was a dancer and never "good" at art. However, when I made my first film I was smitten, and it felt so natural and satisfying to work with a visual medium. And yet when I need energy, I have to move my body, preferably outdoors in nature. To recuperate I close my eyes and listen to the sound of the wind, the bird calls, my dog howling with the fire engine (he does that, maybe that's his creative DNA). My least used perception is conceptual (maybe you already guessed that) and this book is demanding that I build my conceptual muscles… Interestingly, I am very structured and get pleasure in creating forms and can easily contain a large group. But when my husband, who is conceptual and brilliant, describes his latest intricate idea, I have to work hard to follow, and often I realize I'm watching how the sunlight plays across his face and how the shadows form on the floor…and then I have to ask him to start again…

CHAPTER 4

Stages of Creative Process

In a small room at a major children's hospital, four very experienced health professionals and I were sitting around a large table. They were all looking at me very intently and waiting for an explanation as to why the patient I was seeing was spending session after session making hands of varying shapes and sizes. I told them the story she chose was "The Handless Maiden," but at this they rolled their eyes. And I proudly stated that this homeless adolescent who never followed up with any appointments was showing up regularly each week. At this they seemed a little more impressed, but still skeptical. The psychiatrist asked about confronting childhood issues, the psychologist asked about changes in behaviors, the social worker asked about living conditions, and the medical doctor asked about her health. After an uncomfortable silence, I patiently explained the stages of creative process and said that she was in the immersion stage and that this was necessary for insight. Surprisingly, they all nodded their heads and seemed to understand. I realized that by presenting a different framework and speaking the language of creativity rather than one they were familiar with, I had allowed all of them to enter a different paradigm for healing (it also got me off the hook).

According to the *Cambridge Online Dictionary*, to "create" means to "bring into being, to cause to exist, to form, to produce." Each time we sit down to play an instrument, compose a poem, or paint on canvas, we are bringing something new into the world. It doesn't matter if there is an audience. What matters is that we have taken the time and space to honor our creative voice. Even though we may have played the same scales on the piano for years, it will be a little different each time.

That is the unique quality and paradox of creativity that we must be fully committed to the unknown. We need to maintain curiosity and openness on the one hand and almost obsessive perseverance on the other. Yet this paradox is what keeps us healthy since we are full of conviction yet also full of doubt. "Maybe I won't get through the scales today, I'll make a mistake, but I am determined to practice anyway…" Commitment is healthiest when it exists despite doubt, so that we maintain a sense of balance. Rollo May (1980/1994), an existential psychologist, suggests that this balance is achieved by merging the qualities of two Greek gods: Apollo, the god of light, form, reason, and rational order, and Dionysus, the god of letting go, chaos, surging vitality, and drunkenness. Rosemary Gordon (1978/2018), a Jungian analyst, views this chaos and order in terms of when we engage and let go of our ego. She believes there is a clear demarcation of when the ego is active and when it is passive during the stages of creative process. According to Gordon we need our ego when we begin and when we end, but in the middle, while we are immersed in the act of creativity, we must let the ego go so it does not inhibit us by self-judgment, criticism, and distracting thoughts.

Mihaly Csikszentmihalyi (1990, 2015), a Hungarian-American psychologist, proposed that when we create, we enter a state of "flow." In this state we are highly focussed and clear of distractions or thoughts of failure. We have immediate feedback to our actions, and we are fully in the present moment. According to Csikszentmihalyi, being creative affects the way we live and encourages flexibility in our thinking so that we can find unique and diverse solutions to our problems (Csikszentmihalyi, 2015). While this notion of creativity as a state of "flow" is indeed an integral part of the creative process, there is also another and more challenging aspect. As we face the canvas, the empty studio, the piano, we also face ourselves in whatever state we happen to be in. All our insecurities and vulnerabilities can come to the forefront and sometimes this even stops us from continuing. The potential for "flow" is always there but so is the necessity for destruction. As Picasso states, "Every act of creation is first of all an act of destruction." In the creative process and in our personal development, as some new insight, new perspective, new creation, is struggling to be born, our old habits, thoughts, and patterns must die. Therefore, even as the act of creation can bring us immense joy, it can also be painful. In our growth and urge to find new meaning and creative expression we can also feel guilt since we are shaking up the old self and our old relationship to the world. When we create, we are also searching for meaning, and as our hands shape the clay, or our mouths sing a note, we try and find the essence and significance of what we are doing. The act may be simple; however, the impact can be enormous as we embody both new life and death at the same time. The challenge is always to trust that what we create will take us somewhere new, someplace we have never been before, but exactly where we need to go.

The stages of creative process that I use in the *Story Within* are: Preparation; Immersion; Incubation; Illumination; and Verification. These stages are based on several different models (Botella, Zenasni, and Lubart, 2018) and my own clinical and teaching experience. I have found that providing an outline of the different stages and steps in the creative process is helpful as you go through the *Story Within*. These same stages can also be a framework for the therapeutic process and for personal development. Even though it is never a straight line and the stages can blur and occur simultaneously, it is important to understand the qualities of each stage. Of course, culture can and does impact on creativity and I realize that these stages that I propose may not be applicable nor relevant for every culture and community. Therefore, please make modifications and adjustments so that it makes sense for your specific context and culture.

1. Preparation

Before we set out on any new adventure, we look at the map, get good strong boots, and pray for good weather. We really have no idea what we will encounter, but we set out anyway. We trust and hope that we have prepared enough that we will be safe no matter what happens. Safety is essential and especially when we are traveling into the inner depths of our own psyche and creativity. To be able to explore our own process we need to ensure that we have set up a safe container in which the depth work can be done. In practical terms, this means that we need to set up a space, decide on a day and time, and get supplies. This is the stage when we commit ourselves to the journey ahead.

The Studio

To create, you need to have a designated space where you can feel free to move, get messy, and make noise. It does not have to be anything fancy, or expensive, just an area where you can keep some creative supplies. Sometimes you can find a community space where you have a locker for storage, or a basement in someone's house who is willing to be the "host" for a group of people going through the process.

Supplies

You need to get some basic creative supplies that will allow you to explore your creativity with different mediums. They don't have to be elaborate, but you need to ensure that you have some basic art materials (paint, markers, crayons, colored pencils, pastels, paper, clay, glue, brushes, etc.), a few percussion instruments (small drums, shakers, blocks, or you can also use pots and pans), fabric (different materials, can even be old sheets, bedspreads, blankets), and other props (rope, wire, nails, straw, boxes). The fun part (budget permitting) is to go to thrift stores, dollar stores, and art, musical, and fabric stores and explore what you are drawn to. A large part of the process is developing trust in your intuition to guide you to exactly what you need, even if you have no idea why. And for your writings, art work, etc., it is essential to have a journal. This can be a notebook you have lying around, your computer or iPad, even your phone (see more details on supplies in Chapter 7, "How to Go Through the Steps").

Schedule

You also need to establish a schedule. One or two times a week is best with a minimum of one hour for each session. You want to allow enough time to explore the creative mediums, go through the steps, and write in your journal.

Circle of Support

Before you enter the process of the *Story Within*, you need to set up a strong container to ensure that you are safe. One way of doing this is to have another professional therapist (creative arts therapist, counselor, psychologist, community worker) who will support you on this inner journey. Or you can find individuals among your friends and colleagues to be a circle of support. It is best if all of the members of this circle are going through the *Story Within* at the same time. This way you can support each other throughout the process and ensure that all members are safe (for specific details about this, please see the witnessing section in Chapter 5, "Therapeutic Frame," and also Chapter 7, "How to Go Through the Steps").

2. Immersion

Once we have gathered our creative supplies, set up the therapeutic space, and found our circle of support, we are ready to dive into the first two *Story Within* exercises, *The Encounter* and *Chaos and Order*. In these exercises we explore the mediums, play with materials, discover our own creative DNA, and enter the unknown. There is a trust in the process itself and in the wisdom of the arts to lead us where we need to go. This can be a wonderful time, almost childlike, full of play and rediscovery of being immersed in the arts. As we go through the next three exercises, *Finding and Telling the Story*, *Making a Mask*, and *Placing and Embodying the Mask*, we enter the world of our chosen character and this can lead us directly into our own unconscious. As we move deeper into the immersion stage during these exercises, along with the sense of enjoyment and creative expression can come feelings of being muddled or confused. We can find ourselves repeating the same images, movements, or writings over and over without a sense of meaning. This can be challenging, bringing discomfort and a sense that we are stuck, or blocked. It is during this stage that our own inner demons appear and challenge us. Often this can be painful, and we want to give up. It is essential to allow this stage to take its time and to trust that even though we may not know where we are headed, even though we are suffering, something is working and leading us.

This underground, and unconscious, immersion is necessary for true creativity and personal growth. When we enter the sixth step of the process, *Finding the Moment,* it is often a pivotal time, leading us to the essence of what the character and story are trying to tell us. This can be both illuminating and overwhelming and sometimes we need to step back and take a break.

3. Incubation

At some point near the end of the immersion stage it feels like we cannot go on, nothing makes sense, and our creativity feels stilted and dead. This is when we enter the incubation stage and need to let it all go. This stage is the one where you might go for a long hike, read a great novel, or sing loudly in the shower. The point is to take a break from the process and stop consciously thinking or focussing on your creativity or your character. It is important to let go of our conscious way of working so that the unconscious has time and space to find its own solutions. By letting our minds wander, we are truly incubating, and even though we may feel as if we are doing nothing, all our creativity is percolating and then miraculously leads to new insights and discoveries.

4. Illumination

Out of the inner work in the immersion stage and the unconscious percolation of the incubation stage comes illumination as we enter the next five steps of the process: *Soundscape, Environment, Directing Someone Else, Finding the Obstacle and Helper,* and *The Edge.* It is often in these exercises that insight happens, a sudden yet holistic new understanding and breakthrough around a central issue in our life. We cannot force it, however much we try. Real insight does not come from a conscious decision but rather emerges gradually and on its own. Often this experience of insight or illumination occurs against what we consciously hold on to, and yet there is an accompanying certainty, a sense of absolute knowing or inner truth. There is a vividness to the experience and a sense that our relationship to the world has changed. These insights come at a cost—we must face our inner demons and challenges and be willing to be vulnerable. Just when we feel the most uncovered, the most raw, something miraculous happens and there is an opening, a sense of ease and profound gratitude for what we have discovered. Insight will happen at various times for each one of us and during different steps of the process. For some it is through the art, for others the drama, for someone else while walking down the street. The connection with our character leads us to a deep and immediate understanding about some issue in our life. Sadly, we cannot control when insight happens, but as we immerse ourselves in our creativity and in our character this process emerges gradually and in its own time. Our hidden and inaccessible inner stories and narratives are revealed, and we are changed.

5. Verification

As a last step we need to find a way to verify and ground our new insights, discoveries, and new way of being, into the day-to-day world. The last exercise, *Final Presentation/Ritual,* is a time for reflection and analysis about what has emerged during the process. We look over all our creations and our journal and notice the patterns, the moments of insight, and when they occurred. What might have seemed random in terms of dreams, conversations, chance meetings, and creative mistakes now takes on a new meaning and starts to make sense. It is in this stage that we learn why we chose our story and character and how it relates to our own life. The hidden story, the one buried deep in our unconscious, can come to light and now we understand more about who we are. Throughout the process we came to live the reality of our character's journey and found ourselves confronting our character's trauma or deepest fear which we now realize was our own. We are ready to share our discoveries with our circle of support and perhaps others through a structured presentation/ritual (for details see the last step in the process of the *Final Presentation/Ritual* exercise). This can involve a small performance, writings, music, art piece, dance, or ritual, any form that truly expresses our journey with our story and character. This last stage is meant to be a way of closure for you and for your circle of support that is like a rite of passage.

Stages of the Creative Process as a Therapeutic Frame

The above stages of creative process can also be used as a therapeutic frame for both the therapist and the client. Having a basic understanding of each stage of the creative process can be especially useful as an alternative or complementary way of viewing the process of therapy. It can also be a new and perhaps more open and creative way of discussing the progression of our clients with other professionals without the limitations and often narrow descriptions in the medical model.

1. Preparation

CLIENTS

For the client some aspect of their lives feels out of control or is causing suffering, and the decision to seek help is the beginning of the preparation stage. When clients enter the therapy room for the first time, they are testing the waters, wondering if this person can be trusted with their hidden and darkest secrets. They must look within themselves to determine what style of therapy resonates. Once they have made a decision to continue with therapy, they begin the process of becoming aware of their reactions and relationships, and how they respond to the world. This burgeoning awareness of their own habitual patterns and the way these patterns interfere with their own wellbeing can become a motivation for change. Their willingness to accept the idea that things need to change is an integral part of completing the preparation stage.

THERAPIST

We as therapists need to prepare ourselves for working with a new and unique person. This preparation can take many forms; however, it is essential that we have some ritual or practices that allow us to clear our minds of assumptions and bias so that we can be truly open to the person before us. And we need to build our psychic and physical energy for the journey ahead so we can be a strong and stable support. This is the time when we discover the client's unique verbal and creative language, set up a structure, and commit to working together.

2. Immersion
CLIENTS

The next step is to immerse themselves in the process of therapy. In creative arts therapies the client starts to engage with the different creative mediums. In verbal therapy this can be when they start to bring important aspects of their life into the sessions. They begin to understand that they cannot solve their problem totally with their rational mind. Questioning their belief systems, and habitual ways of responding, become central and necessary. Out of this develops a curiosity about their own unconscious material and a sense that something new and unexpected needs to come through. This is when dreams and personal symbols and metaphors enter the therapy. It is in the immersion stage that clients really begin to discover and uncover important aspects of their own hidden story.

THERAPIST

For the therapist the immersion stage is when they become cognizant of the client's unique unconscious language, metaphors, and themes. As these powerful symbols emerge for the first time the therapist needs to be alert and pay close attention, not only to the client but also to their own responses to what is brought into the sessions. It is particularly important that the therapist ensure that they do not have an agenda at this stage, that they remain open and curious without interfering with the client's own process. When unconscious material is seen for the first time it is a very tentative and fragile state for the client, and any strong direction or interpretation from the therapist can strongly influence and perhaps destroy the process. The goal for the therapist is to provide safe and strong containment for these emerging discoveries and unconscious material.

3. Incubation
CLIENTS

At this stage the client, who has been working hard and has faced difficult aspects of themselves, needs to take a break. They may want to stop therapy for a while, take a vacation, or focus on something less demanding. This is an important process to let the conscious mind relax and get out of the way so the unconscious can work on its own.

THERAPIST
For the therapist this can be a challenging stage since it can appear that the client is withdrawing, and the therapy is not progressing. It is helpful if the therapist understands the stages of creative process so that they can offer support for the client's incubation without adding unnecessary anxiety or interference.

4. *Illumination*
CLIENTS
For clients this is an exciting and demanding stage when insights begin to arise spontaneously. Connections are made between aspects of their daily lives and their unconscious material, symbols, and metaphors. While insights can be liberating, they are also challenging the habitual and familiar ways of being. This tension and struggle between the old and the new can cause anxiety and sometimes even a profound sense of loss or mourning.

THERAPIST
The therapist needs to be aware of the inherent struggle within the illumination stage so they can assist clients as they navigate these difficult waters. Sometimes the therapist can be so excited by the client's new insights that they fail to acknowledge the tension and anxiety the client is feeling about letting go of their destructive yet familiar patterns of behavior. It is important for therapists to equally honor the new emergent insights and discoveries, and the potential sense of loss and mourning for the old familiar habits and ways of being.

5. *Verification*
CLIENTS
The final stage for clients is a time to integrate insights and discoveries from the therapy sessions into daily life. Before they can do this, they need to create a closing ritual to acknowledge their process. The verification comes from sharing this closing ritual with others so that

their internal process is communicated within an external creative form. This serves as a rite of passage showing that they are now ready to "graduate" from the therapy.

Therapist

For the therapist it is essential they help the client to determine the appropriate format for the closing ritual that will truly express the client's journey. In addition, the therapist needs to prepare themselves for letting go of the client. As therapists we become attached to our clients and need a ritual for ourselves to say goodbye and honor our own learning and work with this individual.

> I am definitely in the preparation stage…gathering the words and materials to create a book, trusting that, somehow, I can convey what is most important, the essence of my work over the past 20 years. Part of me wonders if this is possible to truly connect with you, the reader, when we won't see each other, when I won't have the pleasure of witnessing your creative offerings… It takes great faith to begin a new journey, and both of us will have to trust that we are being called and there is a story and character waiting in the wings (and perhaps with wings) to enter our lives…

CHAPTER 5

Therapeutic Frame

I had just moved to Montreal from the United States and was hired to work as a creative arts therapist on a psychiatric unit of a major hospital. During my initial interview I was asked if I spoke French and I said, "No." However, when I arrived to lead my first group of inpatients diagnosed with schizophrenia, I was shocked to discover that they only spoke French. Desperate, I decided maybe if I spoke English very loudly and slowly, they would understand. Of course, this was not successful, and for the rest of the session I used a lot of mime and hand gestures. Somehow, we managed to communicate based on the kindness and patience of the group. Over the course of the next few sessions I brought my French dictionary with me and tried to string words together to form cohesive sentences. However, I believe I mostly said things like "chair, move, here, now." The group was very attentive (because they never knew what would come out of my mouth) and really tried to help, offering suggestions. One day when I felt I had mastered enough French to feel more comfortable, I was leading them in a relaxation exercise and I said, "Relaxez les jambons." They were lying on the floor and several lifted their heads and asked "les jambons?" and I proudly stated, "Oui, les jambons." Noticing that everyone looked very confused and some were trying hard not to laugh, I looked in my dictionary and realized I had asked them to "relax their hams." The word for legs in French is "les jambes" and the word for ham is "les jambons." I started to laugh and then all of us were rolling on the floor laughing and saying "Relaxez les jambons" over and over. The fact that I could laugh at my own ignorance and foolishness allowed all of us to share a precious moment of vulnerability and closeness. For the group, this was a turning point when a real alliance was built. From then on

> when a patient was stuck, or we reached a tough moment, someone would inevitably say "Relaxes les jambons" and we would laugh and remember that moment and something would ease. For me, this was a huge lesson as to what "healing" and "therapy" means. I realized that the best I could offer was my full presence with all my foolishness and imperfections and that this allowed them to relax and not feel that they had to be perfect. And perhaps most importantly, I realized that therapy is always about learning a new language. We cannot possibly know what specific words or metaphors mean for our clients and we must be open to admitting we do not know and enjoy the process of stumbling and making mistakes…

What does it mean to be a therapist? While techniques, literature, schools, and training programs abound, it is difficult to pinpoint exactly how to "help" someone else. "Healing" is a commonly used term and yet there is no agreement on the definition. The concept remains confusing and inexact. Perhaps this is as it should be, since the body/mind/spirit is so unique for each person. For me, the process of "healing" inspires awe and humility. When we enter a person's life at their most vulnerable, in a way it is a form of prayer. It does not have to do with a belief system or religion, but there is always a surrendering to something larger. How can I possibly know what is right for someone else? I do not. No one really knows what experience anyone else should be having. All we can do is accompany, be fully present, and offer to hold space, so that another person can discover their own internal world. For the *Story Within* approach there are some essential guidelines that will be helpful in going through the process. I believe that developing these essential skills helps us to learn the unique language of our clients, those we witness, and of our own unconscious. Many of these skills will be familiar for any therapist; however, there are also specific skills necessary for this particular approach. I have also included questions for each skill set to determine if this approach is right for you, your clients, or members of your circle of support.

Some of the words in the questions may not make sense for diverse cultures and communities. Please find your own words and cultural context that make sense but keep the question open and allow time and space for the person or yourself to respond.

Compassion, Empathy, Imperfection

> When we feel empathy for another person but then can also feel that we can be helpful, we are less likely to burn out.

In the helping profession we are often told to "feel empathy" and "be compassionate" and yet we are also advised to put up boundaries and make sure not to "burn out." This double message can cause confusion, and in response we sometimes try to play a role as the "helper," with a set expression, posture, and tone of voice. We all play roles and take on personas, as a way of negotiating various aspects of our lives. We are mother, father, son, daughter, sibling, friend, professional, lover, and many others. Role playing can be fun and necessary; however, in terms of truly meeting the "other" or finding an authentic place of connection, it can get in the way. What is compassion? How do we truly empathize with another person? Is there a difference between empathy and compassion? According to several researchers, compassion is not the same as empathy even though the concepts are related and often used interchangeably (Cummings et al., 2018; Lim and DeSteno, 2016). Our ability to take the perspective of and viscerally feel the emotions of another person is referred to as empathy. There are actual "mirror neurons" that arise automatically when we witness someone in pain. While compassion is literally defined as "to suffer together," it is expressed when those feelings of empathy include the desire to help (Lim and DeSteno, 2016). An important distinction between feeling empathy and compassion is how they can affect our overall wellbeing. If we are frequently feeling the pain of someone else, it may become overwhelming, especially if we feel helpless. This is a widespread problem for caregivers and health providers and has been labeled as "burnout" or "empathy fatigue." Compassion, however, is a renewable resource. When we feel empathy for another person but then also feel that we can be helpful, we are less likely to burn out.

Another reason compassion may boost our wellbeing is that it can help broaden our perspective beyond ourselves. Some recent studies have even suggested that compassion and empathy employ different regions of the brain and that compassion can combat empathetic distress (Chierchia and Singer, 2017; Costa and Costa, 2016; Seppälä et al., 2017). So, it seems that for anyone in the helping professions it would be important to develop compassion. We not only need compassion for others but also for ourselves. And for those engaging with the *Story Within,* the overarching container of compassion for ourselves and others is the basic ingredient for creating safety, connection, and depth.

To be helpful as a therapist or witness we must be open to the other person's reality and state of being. If we are someone who moves easily in the world, it might be hard to truly empathize with someone who struggles just to say hello in a social gathering. And yet we all have a place of fear inside, we all have wounds, seen and unseen. Embracing our own wounds and discomfort helps us to empathize and feel compassion for someone else. Once we feel compassion, though, how do we know how to be "helpful"? One simple way is the act of listening with our full presence. This can be one of the most compassionate and helpful acts we can offer. Unfortunately, with technology and our busy lives, compassionate listening has become increasingly rare. It is not only listening to the words but making a full visceral connection that tells the other person that they are valuable, and worthy of our full attention. Compassionate listening requires us to not only feel empathy for the other person's suffering, but also to trust in the other person's capacity for self-healing. This trust in an innate desire in all of us towards health and wellbeing is the essence of compassion. It takes away the sense that we are responsible for someone else's healing. We are not. All we can do is listen and be fully present so that we can respond authentically in a way that meets the other person where they are. In this place of authentic meeting, transformation and healing can occur. For engaging with the *Story Within* there are ways to develop our skills to be a more compassionate presence and listener. The first is to become aware of what gets in the way of our empathy and compassion. Can we feel the fears and dreams of those who are in political opposition to our own beliefs? Is there a place of meeting with those who hold what we might consider extreme adherence to a religion or set of values? How do we hold both the perpetrator and victim in our hearts? None of this is easy and all of us struggle, yet the act of becoming aware and honestly confronting our own bias, prejudice, and blind spots can offer a way to developing more open compassion. Another way is to practice open listening: letting go of any "role" we play, any agenda or sense that we must prove or be anything, and just allow for a pure connection. It can be helpful to begin this practice with colleagues or those where the relationship is simple and less complicated and then progress to loved ones. We can also practice this on public transportation, when we sit next to others. Can we sit together in compassion, without words or outward communication, resting in a larger sense of compassion that holds us all?

Question

What does compassion mean for you, and how do you experience this? Are there people in your life who you have trouble feeling compassion for, and is this something you would like to develop?

> If the answer is only one word, or there is no real interest in speaking about this, then this may not be the right approach. However, if there is interest, and a sense of curiosity and willingness to explore personal bias and blind spots to develop more open compassion, then it makes sense to go to the next step.

Comfort and Ability to Work with Story, Myth, and Metaphor

> A mythic perspective can teach us to be more open and curious about what we encounter every day.

There are many ways to approach healing and working with personal issues and challenges. The *Story Within* uses a mythic frame of reference. What this means is that instead of discussing or approaching a problem directly, the focus is on finding and working with a specific story and character. Therefore, both the therapist and client must be willing and able to work with metaphor and symbol. Currently, we live in an information age, with quick access via the internet to all the facts we need for whatever purpose we decide. However, the subtle language of metaphor and symbol has been pushed aside or coerced in the service of advertising or a specific belief system. To work with story, it is necessary to have a basic understanding of what metaphor and symbol mean. A metaphor compares two things that are not similar and shows that they do have something in common. It comes from the Greek *metapherein*, meaning "transference." A word or phrase denoting one kind of object is used in place of another to suggest a likeness or analogy between them (*Cambridge Online Dictionary*). As Aristotle (384–322 BCE) stated, "Metaphor consists in giving the thing a name that belongs to something else." Whereas a symbol is anything that stands for, or represents, something else. Symbolism is the practice or art of using an object, word, person, place, or action to represent something significant and deeper than its literal meaning. Both metaphor and symbol are inherent in myths, fairy tales, and traditional stories, and in working with them we connect to a mythic consciousness and our inner world. To be able to work with the *Story Within* process in a consistent and effective way we must have the ability to think abstractly and symbolically. Therefore, there are some groups I would not recommend for this approach. Those with Alzheimer's, dementia, or major cognitive impairments will not be the best candidates. To sustain a long-term symbolic projection, memory must be coherent and consistent. There are many other effective techniques for working with these groups. Also, this approach is not recommended for those with active psychosis or delusions since they can struggle with discerning reality and it may not be helpful to encourage a long-term projection onto a fictional character. Also, those with autism spectrum disorder may not be able to work abstractly with metaphor and symbol and may be best served with an approach that is more concrete. Other than the above populations, anyone can be a candidate.

Even if we do not have a history of reading or working with stories, we can develop the skills to learn to trust the inherent healing within the stories themselves. To do this we need to read or listen to a variety of different myths, fairy tales, and traditional stories, preferably from diverse cultures, and in their original form. Unfortunately, Disney and others have sanitized these stories to such a degree that the darker and essential elements are missing. I would suggest searching on the internet, in bookstores, and in libraries. There is something wonderful and timeless about sitting in a comfortable chair in a library, getting lost in a book of stories. We can also find them in audio books or podcasts. You may want to experiment with reading and listening and noticing if you respond differently depending how the story is presented. As we read or listen to the stories, we open our minds to allow the metaphors and symbols to enter our unconscious. Without judgment or analysis, we become familiar with some of the archetypal themes, patterns, challenges, and narrative structures. This familiarity helps us to develop a mythic sense that there is a larger meaning and significance to the way we live our lives. We identify with the fictional protagonists as they face obstacles, battle inner and outer demons, and find mentors and helpers along the way. A mythic perspective can teach us to be more open and curious about what we encounter every day. Instead of responding to our challenges as a victim, we can become empowered to face these trials as part of a larger and personally meaningful narrative.

Question

Are there any stories or novels, TV shows, or films you like? If so, please describe in detail what it is about this story or a character that touches you.

> If the answer is only one word, or there is no real interest in speaking about this, then this may not be the right approach. However, if there is interest, and a sense of identification with a story or character and an ability to connect to the character, then it makes sense to go to the next step.

Comfort with No Interpretation, No Agenda, Entering the Unknown

"Having no destination,
I am never lost."

Ikkyū Sōjun, Buddhist monk and poet (1394–1481)

Embrace discomfort as a friend or teacher…

For therapy to be effective and long-lasting, clients need to come to understand their personal issues and material in their own time and within their own personal framework. If we as therapists impose our own agenda and interpretation, this can interfere with the therapeutic process, particularly when the client is in a fragile place, struggling to uncover hidden and inaccessible parts of themselves. The therapist must be willing to enter "the unknown" along with their clients. As Daniel J. Siegal (2007) suggests, it is only in a healthy state of uncertainty that we can truly discover something new. When we are certain, we don't feel the need to pay attention. In contrast, when we are uncertain, we become more sensitive to context and engage in the present and can come up with more creative solutions (Binder, Martin, and Schwind, 2018; Siegal, 2007). As therapists this willingness to "not know" helps us be more present for our clients as they gradually discover their own sense of knowing, creative DNA, meaning making, insights, and transformation. The symbols and metaphors in the chosen story will have a unique and significant meaning for each person. However, the meaning and significance cannot be apparent or obvious at the beginning as this would limit and stop the process. If we choose a story and character based on what we already know then we will not discover anything new. In contrast, we will only be reinforcing our habitual ways of thinking and feeling. This is common and is why so many people who have been in therapy for years do not really make progress or change. Habits are comfortable even if they cause suffering. Our brain will automatically follow the familiar neuropathways that we have used over and over (Levin, 2018). To counter this, we must find avenues that are not familiar or habitual.

Working with story and metaphor can offer something different. If we choose a story and character with a sense of resonance that is not understood and elicits some sense of discomfort, then we can truly enter a process of discovery. It is the gradual uncovering of meaning that allows for real change.

To benefit from going through the *Story Within* process, and for the therapist or witness to be helpful, it is necessary to develop the skills to be comfortable in the "unknown." To do this we must become as aware as possible of our internal voices and fears. Often it is fear that keeps us from being fully open and present. Even though we know this intellectually, the challenge is to build the skills to be able to sit with fear and embrace our discomfort. After all, without discomfort, growth cannot happen. One of the ways to build these skills is to set a time every day for 10–20 minutes of silent meditation and reflection. The goal is to develop a sense of open awareness without attachment to thoughts, narratives, or belief systems. What are we without our thoughts? What happens when we rest in silence? Begin with a gentle focus on the breath and notice where in your body you feel tension. Without judgment, or feeling you must change or do anything, just pay attention to what is happening within your inner landscape. What are the thoughts, emotions, tensions, that rise to the surface? Can you let them emerge as if they are just part of a landscape, forming trees, clouds, rivers, all within the vast open space of the "unknown"? This can be challenging as our mind will want to focus on something and create a narrative. Once that happens, we have left the "unknown" and set up a "known" or familiar story line that distracts us from what is present right now. Often there is a fear of silence and of not controlling our experience by our thoughts and familiar interpretations. Paradoxically, we all know that, ultimately, we have little control over anything. We have no idea what will happen next, but we like to think we do. So, in this exercise it is about developing more comfort in resting in the "unknown."

Once you have become grounded in this practice then take it to the next step, which is to observe what comes up when you are with others. How does the interaction affect your postures, tension, breathing, thoughts, and feelings? If you feel discomfort, how do you respond to it? Do you disconnect from yourself, become agitated or angry, run away from the person or situation? It is essential as therapists that we learn about our personal response to discomfort and develop the muscles to sit with it and even embrace it as a friend or teacher. The more we can observe within our own internal process, the less we will project our own uncomfortable feelings onto others. Is it possible to maintain a sense of "not knowing" and curiosity when in relationship? What happens if we become more open to the unexpected even in familiar relationships? Resting in the "unknown" while in the world changes our relationship to it. Another simple exercise for developing the ability to be comfortable with the unknown is to go for a walk (outside or inside) and alternate walking with a sense of knowing what is in front of you with a stance of curiosity and not knowing. What changes in your body/mind/spirit when you approach what is in front of you without a sense of knowing what it is? Can you become genuinely curious with a sense of play and openness? This may be the same tree you pass every day, but what if you stop and see it as if you have never seen it before, as if it could be anything, maybe even not a tree? Can you notice the texture, the shapes, the colors, and your own response without labeling or "knowing" what it is? Playing with this exercise can be helpful in gaining more comfort with the unknown and can help to change how we approach our loved ones, our clients, and ourselves. It is often the label we place on someone that can limit how we see them and how we interact.

Question

Are there any times in your life when you have let yourself surrender fully to the "unknown" and, if so, when was this and how did it feel? It could be when listening to music, engaging in a creative act, lovemaking, or exploring nature.

> If the answer is "never" and there is no interest in reflecting on this, then this may not be the right approach. However, if there is interest, and a sense of curiosity and reflection about what it means to be in the "unknown," then it makes sense to continue.

Comfort with the Creative Process

> It is through a creative response that we learn to trust the unconscious…

The *Story Within* approach is based on using creativity as an essential therapeutic tool. Working with diverse mediums we engage in a creative projection onto a chosen story and character. Therefore, it is essential for the therapist and anyone working with this approach to have a sense of comfort and openness to the creative process. This does not mean in any way that we must be an artist or be skilled in any or all mediums. However, it does mean that we are willing to explore our own creativity and, as Miss Frizzle from *The Magic School Bus* says, "Get Messy!!" (Cole and Degen, 1994/2001). We cannot expect our clients to try a new creative medium if we are not willing to do so ourselves. We may be comfortable with one creative medium, for example singing or drawing; perhaps we sang in a choir, or maybe we liked drawing as a child. The challenge is to engage in mediums we are not comfortable or skilled in. Often this lack of technique allows us to engage in a more exploratory and open way. Since we are not skilled, we don't have the same expectations that we will produce something "perfect." In contrast, we can enter the unknown and explore in a more free and vulnerable manner. If as a therapist we are willing to model this vulnerability and being "imperfect" by engaging with mediums we are not skilled at, it frees our clients to let go of their own inner critic and expectations.

Art-to-Art Response

One of the techniques that is integral to the *Story Within* is the art-to-art response. In therapy we often use reflection to create a therapeutic alliance and to help the client feel heard and supported. Reflection does not need to be verbal to be effective. In art-to-art response, instead of reflecting verbally we give a reflection through a creative medium. This allows a sense of immediacy, vulnerability, and communication that would be impossible to achieve through words alone.

In individual sessions it can initiate a much stronger therapeutic alliance since the therapist is seen as human and gives an authentic creative response. It also takes away a sense of power difference and inequality, letting the client see the vulnerability and creative offering from the therapist or witness. It can be greatly beneficial for the therapist to respond creatively through a medium that they are not proficient in. This models risk taking, vulnerability, and imperfection and can be very therapeutic for clients. When done in the group it creates a powerful sense of group cohesion and allows members to bond in a much more authentic and intimate way. Clients learn how to communicate and respond to each other in a non-judgmental and non-interpretive manner. They learn to communicate from their own honest experience as expressed creatively rather than an intellectual analysis or interpretation. It is through the art-to-art responses that members of a group come together to develop closeness, take greater risks, and trust that they can support each other. For everyone it can be empowering to know that by responding authentically from our own experience we can have an impact and be helpful for someone else. Knowing that the response will be creative rather than verbal encourages a distinct way of listening. As a listener we pay attention without feeling we must give advice, an interpretation, or an analysis. We bring our full sense of presence and openness and then respond with an honest expression of what touched and moved us in the hope that it will offer something useful.

How can we develop more comfort with the creative process and diverse mediums? How can we learn to trust the arts enough so that we feel comfortable responding creatively instead of, or in addition to, verbally? There are several techniques for developing these skills. For the *Story Within* approach it is helpful to combine learning about stories with learning how to be more creative. After reading a new myth, fairy tale, or traditional story, instead of an analysis or interpretation, make a drawing or a movement, or compose a song or a poem. It does not have to be anything elaborate or time consuming and need not conform to any standards of beauty or perfection. This is your response, your creative voice. All that matters is that it is authentic and, in some way, expresses what touched you about the story. If you feel uncomfortable about your drawing skills, make a collage with images from magazines or play a percussive instrument and make sounds. You don't need to be skilled in the medium to be expressive. This is not a performance, and no one needs to see your responses. It is only for you to develop your creative muscles and become more comfortable responding with diverse artistic mediums. It is through a creative response that we learn to trust the unconscious. If we can trust this process, then we can guide others to trust their own unconscious and allow the story and character to lead them where they need to go.

Question

Have you ever sung in the shower, doodled in long meetings, danced to the radio when no one was around? Can you remember exploring creatively as a child, and if so, what do you remember?

> If the answer is "never" and there is no interest in reflecting on this, then this may not be the right approach. However, if there is interest, and a sense of curiosity and reflection about what it means to be creative, then it makes sense to continue.

The Power of Being a Witness and Containment

> The presence of the outer witness can become a model of compassion that eventually becomes internalized in the person being witnessed.

The role of the witness is an essential aspect of the *Story Within* approach. Having a witness provides safety and a sense of order and containment for the chaos and uncertainty of the process. When I work with clients individually, I am always in the role of a witness even though I may engage in creative activities or responses to help the client. When done in the context of a group I am the main and consistent witness, thus providing a consistent container for the group. The other participants also act as witnesses during certain exercises. This builds up the capacity for them to learn how to be an effective witness or listener. As the therapist I set up the structure and guide clients through each stage of the process, providing a strong container within which clients feel safe to allow difficult personal material to emerge. I never choose the story, character, or moment for the client, but, rather, support the client in this essential and therapeutic process.

What does it mean to be a witness? Are there specific skills that need to be developed? My understanding and experience of being a witness was highly influenced by my training and work with Janet Adler (2002, 2015). She is a pioneer in the field of Authentic Movement, an improvisational movement practice done with eyes closed and in the presence of one or more witnesses. The idea is to follow the spontaneous impulses of the body and let go of judgment. The witness watches and notices her own inner responses to the mover. First initiated by Mary Whitehouse (in 1958), it was Adler (2002, 2015) who developed the role of the witness in the practice of Authentic Movement. As she describes, the witness supports the mover by holding the space and sharing the concentration. Afterwards the mover and the witness exchange their experiences verbally or by drawing, writing, and moving. The presence of the outer witness can become a model of compassion for the mover that gradually becomes internalized (Adler, 2002, 2015).

To follow the steps of the *Story Within* approach it is essential to have someone else there to be a witness and to work with you in several of the creative exercises. If it is feasible, I highly encourage you to have a circle of support made up of other therapists, or professionals, who have a strong interest in self-reflection and engaging in a personal journey. If this is not feasible, or you are concerned about what might emerge, you can do this process as part of your own personal therapy. Having a witness provides a safe container in which you can explore your own internal process. We all know how important it is to have someone there when we are suffering, and how devastating it is to be alone with our pain. As humans we are social animals and need one another to thrive. And while our families and friends provide day-to-day support, when we embark on a deeply personal journey, we need to identify specific individuals who can take on the role of being a witness. This is an essential and significant role that requires a mature sense of being able to be supportive without being intrusive or directive, offering a non-judgmental stance of acceptance for whatever is expressed, and absolute integrity in terms of confidentiality and safety. There needs to be an established sense of trust that this person or group of individuals will be able to hold whatever strong emotions and personal material emerge and will also be able to determine when we need to seek additional professional help.

Becoming a strong witness is really learning about "presence." It is a skill that can be developed with practice. For many of us we take on the "role" of being a "good therapist" or a "good listener": sitting in a particular way and forming an expression that we think will be "healing." While this may be helpful for the therapist to feel in control, it can take away from an authentic therapeutic relationship. The more fully we can inhabit our body/mind/spirit in an honest and open way, the more we can be present for our clients. The same is true for being a witness. As a witness our primary task is to hold space for others in our circle, to listen, watch, and respond in as authentic a way as possible. To do this we need to pay attention to what comes up for us as witnesses—be curious as to when we become under-distanced (overwhelmed by emotion) or over-distanced (distracted and removed from our emotions). What is hard for us to witness in another person? When do we turn away? What subjects make us most uncomfortable: death, sex, suffering, loss? The more we can identify what makes us uncomfortable and stay with the discomfort, the more we can develop our skills as witnesses and the capacity to expand our circumference of what we can contain. Clients will never go to a place that they feel the therapist cannot handle. For example, if a therapist is uncomfortable with death, it will remain taboo in the therapy. The more skills we develop as witnesses, the deeper the personal sharing and expression will be.

There are a few simple exercises I recommend to build our skills as witnesses. The first is to pay attention to your postural stance in your role as therapist or witness. How do you "hold" yourself? Do you have a set expression on your face? What are your arms, legs, shoulders, head, and back doing as you listen? Are you breathing deeply or shallowly? Does all this change depending on who you are with and, if so, in what way? Without judgment or analysis, it is helpful to begin to pay attention to your non-verbal communication and develop a kinesthetic awareness of your body. For some of you, at the beginning, this may be a daunting task with little sense of your muscular tension and holding patterns, but if you practice this and write about your discoveries, you can learn to have a more open and authentic witnessing stance. Once you become aware of a specific expression you habitually use as your "therapist face," you can experiment with altering this to be less imposed and more of who you are. Another exercise is to continue with the silent meditation and reflection exercise for entering the unknown and then go out and just witness random people on the street, in a café, or at a park and pay attention to what comes up for you in terms of your body and emotions. How does what you see affect how you witness? Does your posture or expression change depending on what you see? You are not trying to have a "neutral" expression, or no expression, but rather just gaining awareness so that you are not locked into one way of presenting yourself and witnessing others.

Question
When have you felt that you were truly seen and heard? What were the qualities that allowed for you to feel this way? When did you feel you were not heard or seen and that others imposed their agenda onto you? How did that make you feel?

> If the answer is "never" and there is no interest in reflecting on this, then this may not be the right approach. However, if there is interest, and a sense of curiosity and reflection about what it means to be seen and heard, then it makes sense to continue.

Safety First

Whenever we embark on a new adventure, whether it be physical, psychological, or spiritual, we need to ensure our safety. We check out the best routes, the weather, and our supplies, and plan accordingly. Throughout human history there have always been specific rituals designed to protect the individual who ventured into a potentially unsafe and threatening place. For many traditional communities around the world, the Shaman, or healer, entered a type of spiritual trance to seek wisdom for healing, divining the future, or communicating with the spirits of the dead. The Shaman's role is to help the community feel safe and provide a sense of protection from the elements, disease, starvation, and enemies. However, the Shaman also needs to be safe to enter and return from the spiritual trance. They do this by following specific rituals and practices using masks, rattles, dancing, purification ceremonies, physical manipulation, prayer, and/or healing herbs (Dhungana and Yamphu, 2016; Moss, 2012). Similar rituals to provide safety can be found in diverse religions and cultures. Examples include learning to control emotions and desires, mastering the body in ritual or meditation, acquiring difficult skills (learning a sacred language, memorizing scripture and liturgy), becoming altruistic, controlling dietary and sleep habits, and so on. The aim of all these practices is to ensure that the person entering a mystical realm has the appropriate protection and safety to ensure that they will return unharmed. To work with the *Story Within* it is essential to ensure safety at every stage of the process. When we engage with the unconscious and with archetypal material, it can be powerful and sometimes overwhelming. Therefore, the whole sequence and structure of the *Story Within* was developed to provide safety. The fact that the focus is on creativity and a fictional character and story allows for a sense of distance. The pacing can be slow and gradual, and insight occurs organically without being forced. Each exercise has specific instructions aimed at providing a sense of containment and structure for the personal exploration. Even the words used for the directives have been carefully chosen. It is important that those who enter this process have a solid ego strength and can enter a role, or a creative projection, and also de-role or come out of the projection. Similarly, for the Shamans and those entering mystical states, we need specific rituals for entering the mythic realm and for leaving it. Both the therapist/witness and the clients/participants need to stay safe throughout each step.

What does it mean to be safe? Are there specific skills that need to be developed? For me, the most important skill is to be able to identify and recognize when we are not safe. Often those who have experienced trauma, abuse, or PTSD have difficulty in accessing the appropriate signals from their body notifying them of danger. For someone who was abused as a young child, the world is not safe and people cannot be trusted, and yet the mechanism to survive the abuse was to disconnect from the body so that the organic method to ensure safety was overridden. To counteract this disconnect there needs to be a learned sense of trusting the body and the signals. This can take time. For anyone wanting to explore deep personal material it is essential to identify our own body signals for when we feel unsafe. To do this we can begin by imagining a dangerous activity (skydiving, falling from a tree, encountering a dangerous animal) and while we are imagining this feel our kinesthetic response. What is happening with our breath, our muscles, our heartrate? It doesn't matter what we notice as long as we are beginning to feel the connection between an imagined scenario and our own body's way of signaling danger. Once we have done this for a while, we can take the exercise into the world and notice when we feel similar responses from our body. For some of us it may be constant, or for others only when we are called up to speak publicly, or when someone yells at us, or we see a strange dog. The impetus is not important but rather a growing sense of a kinesthetic relationship to our own safety signals. Once we have identified our own responses then we can also work on relaxation and breathing techniques to counteract inappropriate danger signals. We may be responding as if we are being chased by a tiger but, in fact, we just need to give a speech! Developing the skills to identify and work with our own safety signals is essential so that we can go through the *Story Within* in a safe way.

Question

When have you felt that you were truly safe? What were the qualities that allowed for you to feel this way? When did you feel you were not safe, and how did that make you feel?

> If the answer is "never" and there is no interest in reflecting on this, then this may not be the right approach. If they seem distressed by the question and express feelings of wanting to hurt themselves or

others, it is important to recommend that they seek professional help. However, if there is interest, and a sense of curiosity and reflection about what it means to be safe, then it makes sense to continue.

Open Attention and Direct Intention

We are often told to "pay attention" and that this is required if we want to understand something new. In fact, the whole educational model is based on this idea of attention as an essential part of learning. However, we never examine the meaning or personal experience of attention in a kinesthetic and visceral way. What does "attention" mean? In psychology the most common meaning is the concentration of awareness on some phenomenon to the exclusion of other stimuli. There are, for example, times when an individual has difficulty concentrating attention on a task, a conversation, or a set of events. Whereas for Toni Packer (2007), a meditation teacher, the idea of attention is quite different. For her, attention is a state of listening quietly without expectations or effort, an inner stillness and silence so that the mind can rest in a "simple presence." As therapists and witnesses we need to have the ability both to focus and concentrate on something specific, and to stay open to all that we see, hear, and perceive. As dance movement therapists we learn about the different qualities of movement as a combination of the following categories, each with two possible elements: Space/Focus (Direct or Indirect), Time (Quick or Sustained), Weight (Heavy or Light), and Flow (Bound or Free), as outlined by Ajili, Mallem, and Didier (2018) and Chaiklin and Wengrower (2015). In the *Story Within* approach I developed a way of working with both concentration and open awareness, expanding on Laban's (1975) direct and indirect use of space using the terms "Open Attention" and "Direct Intention." Open Attention is more what Packer (2007) was referring to as the ability to see, hear, and perceive what is in front of us without judgment, expectations, or analysis. However, it is not just an intellectual concept but a lived body experience: all of our senses are open so we feel this openness with our eyes, ears, skin, muscles, posture, and movements. In contrast, Direct Intention is when we respond to something we perceive and focus our attention to concentrate on a specific task. This is when, as therapists, we decide on an intervention or a direction we want to encourage for the client. The transition from Open Attention to Direct Intention is subtle and yet can be experienced in the changes in our senses and in our body. We are no longer open to everything around us but choose one thing to hold our attention and a specific task or direction to follow.

How can we develop these skills in a practical and experiential way? To do this we can start by walking around a room with the idea of Open Attention. Let yourself see everything in the room, hear the sounds, feel your feet on the floor, the air on your skin, your muscles as you move, all of this without judgment, expectation, or a specific focus or task. Just allow yourself to rest in awareness of what is happening moment to moment. Experience this as you move through the room, pick up various objects, and if you are brave, encounter other people. Once you have a strong body sense of this state then slowly transition to Direct Intention. Focus on one object in the room and zero in on it so that nothing else exists but this object. Pick it up and study it so that you see the details of the object but are no longer aware of sounds, the air on your skin, your muscles moving. Then choose a specific direction to go to and feel how your body becomes focussed and leads you. Once you have experienced directing your Intention towards different directions, then based on what you see in the room, decide on a specific task and do it. As you accomplish this task, become aware of the changes in your body. Notice your breathing, your facial expression, your muscles and movements. Play with this transition from Open Attention into Direct Intention and notice how you transition from one to the other. What changes make the transition possible? Once you have a strong sense of these two states then practice the same thing when you are out in the world and in conversation. This can become challenging! See what happens. Developing the skills to identify and work with Open Attention and Direct Intention is essential for becoming a stronger witness, therapist, and participant in the *Story Within* process.

Question

When have you felt that you were in a very open state of mind without expectations or judgments? What allowed for this? When have you felt you were in a state of being extremely focussed on one object or task, and what allowed for this?

> If the answer is "never" and there is no interest in reflecting on this, then this may not be the right approach. However, if there is interest, and a sense of curiosity and reflection about what it means to be in an open state and a focussed state, then it makes sense to continue.

∽

> Since creating the *Story Within* I have gone through the process several times, and many stories and characters, Persephone, the young boy in "The Dragon and the Pearl," the Ugly Duckling, etc., were all helpful and led me to unexplored places inside myself. However, as one of my dear friends pointed out, I never had a therapist or witness who was holding the space and supporting me. Somehow, even though I am a huge advocate of having a witness during the process, I felt I could do it alone. But after reading the words in this chapter I realize that I have missed out on a crucial step. Thankfully, I do have an amazing circle of support, a small group of women I have been meeting with for several years. This time I will include them in my process. I can't wait…

CHAPTER 6

Elements in Myths, Fairy Tales, and Traditional Stories

The room was cast in warm shadows with light filtering in from the leaded glass windows. My grandmother and I were settled on the soft couch and she had the book open to my favorite fairy tale "The Boy and the Three Goats." I wanted the same story every time. My grandmother wrapped her big arms around me and smiled and began to read... As the afternoon light faded, we were lost in an old musty book, turning the pages together...

The vinyl record had a purple center and I was old enough to place it on the record player very carefully and turn out the lights. In the darkness I listened as a male voice slowly read aloud the Greek myths. Alone on my bed I listened to tales filled with gods and goddesses...

In college I was a dancer. For the graduation I was asked to choreograph a dance and I created an outdoor piece based on the descent of Persephone into Hades, using movement and music. I had no idea what I was doing, and an active and friendly dog decided to join in the action. It was chaotic, unpredictable, and utterly thrilling... The audience and the dancers were transported into another world full of magic where anything can happen...

Once upon a time... In the beginning... There once was a... In a far-off land... In a small village... All these phrases can be the start of a myth, fairy tale, or traditional story. We hear those words and we know we are about to enter a different world, one with its own framework, references, and unique cultural lens. Many of us have childhood memories of parents, grandmothers, or other loved ones reading us stories, or making up bedtime tales to help us fall asleep. We may have forgotten the stories, but the memories linger in our unconscious. Or, for those with no childhood experience of being read stories, this feels like a new and foreign territory. And yet, there is something universal and almost atavistic about storytelling. From the earliest times humans have always told stories. Oral storytelling was a way to pass down knowledge, culture, and traditions from generation to generation. Once written down, these stories became part of a cultural heritage that helped us make sense of and navigate our world. As we approach working with the *Story Within*, we need to determine what makes a story archetypal and appropriate for this type of exploration. Not all stories are mythic or archetypal: there are certain elements that need to be present. The narrative must contain a sense of a journey or quest, with obstacles, struggle, and tension that the protagonist goes through to change. In contrast, a fable is a short fictional story, in prose or verse, that is used mainly to illustrate a moral lesson, for example "The Ant and the Grasshopper." In this fable the ant saved food for the winter and the grasshopper did not. The moral is that it is better to prepare for the days ahead. A legend is a narrative of human actions that is considered realistic and takes place within human history. Both fables and legends are included in folktales, stories in the oral tradition handed down between generations. While some fables and legends can be appropriate for the *Story Within*, most are not since the element of a quest is missing.

It is important to have tools with which to assess whether a story fits into a mythic framework and will be useful. The word "myth" originates from the Greek word *mythos*, meaning "word," "tale," or "true narrative," referring not only to how it was transmitted but also to its being rooted in truth. *Mythos* was also closely related to the word *myo*, meaning "to teach" or "to initiate into the mysteries." This is how the word was interpreted by Homer when composing his great works, including *The Iliad*, in which he meant to convey a truth (*Merriam Webster Dictionary*). A myth is a sacred story from the past that may explain the origin of the universe and of life, or it may express its culture's moral values in symbolic and human terms. Myths concern the powerful entities who control the human world and the relationship between those powerful entities and human beings. Myths usually contain specific accounts of gods or superhuman beings involved in extraordinary events or circumstances in a time that is unspecified, but which is understood as existing apart from ordinary human experience. While fairy tales are also symbolic and exist apart from ordinary experience, what makes them different from myths are the elements of the fantastic, the appearance of unicorns, elves, mermaids, gnomes, witches, wizards, and magic. A girl can sleep for a hundred years or a carriage can turn into a pumpkin. Fairy tales occur both in oral and in literary form, and the name "fairy tale" ("*conte de fées*" in French) was first used by Madame d'Aulnoy in the late seventeenth century (Salmon, 2018). Many of today's fairy tales have evolved from centuries-old stories that have appeared, with variations, in multiple cultures around the world. For aboriginal and indigenous cultures, their traditional stories differ from fairy tales and myths in that they are not located in the past or "once upon a time" but rather in a timeless present (Little Bear, 2013; Smith, 2016, 2018). Traditional stories were passed on from generation to generation through oral storytelling, expressing cultural beliefs, values, customs, rituals, and history. There are many diverse aboriginal and indigenous groups across the world, and each have unique stories. However, there are some characters or themes that may be similar such as the theme of creation, the trickster, transformation, animal spirits, and connection to the land. Often these traditional stories are deeply based in nature and rich with the symbolism of the seasons, weather, plants, animals, earth, water, sky, and fire (Little Bear, 2009, 2013).

Each culture has a specific cultural lens and framework. However, as Joseph Campbell (2008, 2011, 2017), writer, mythologist, and scholar, suggested, there are some themes that are cross-cultural and universal. He developed the idea of the *monomyth*, a universal story structure that can be a template of how a character goes through a sequence of stages as part of an important personal journey. Although not every story adheres to the exact same stages, within most myths, fairy tales, and traditional stories, there are some essential elements that make them universal and relevant to our own lives. For Campbell, the template was geared to the idea of the protagonist as a male hero.

Whereas Maureen Murdock (2016), a student of Campbell's work, felt his model failed to address the specific psycho-spiritual journey of contemporary women. She developed a model describing the cyclical nature of the female experience. Bolen (2002, 2004, 2011, 2014), in her seminal book *Goddesses in Every Woman*, provides archetypal female images using Greek goddesses. She presents various aspects of womanhood based on the goddesses that are necessary for the female journey towards self-realization. Additionally, Kathleen Ragan (2009, 2010) edited a book that specifically highlights heroines from around the world. So, this question of gender is important and is reflected by the many recent authors who have reinterpreted myths and fairy tales based on a more feminist viewpoint. While I agree that many of the "heroes" are male, there is certainly a cross-cultural tradition of strong and diverse female protagonists such as Draupadi (Indian), Anath (Canaanite), Hel (Norse), Louhi (Finnish), Itzpapalotl (Aztec), Antigone, Artemis, Athena (Greek), Morrigan (Celtic), Mami Wata (African), Sedna (Inuit), and many, many others. While Campbell and others may have had a heteronormative and gender-specific viewpoint, there are also many stories that feature two-spirited, androgynous, or non-binary gender roles, and/or same sex love, such as Shiva, Arjuna/Brihannala (Hindu mythology), Ishtar (Mesopotamian), Hapi (Egyptian), Shinu No Hafuri and his lover Ama No Hafuri (Japanese), Wahineomo (Polynesian, Hawaiian, and Maori), Mawu-Lisa (African), Ungud (Australian, aboriginal), and Chin (Maya and Aztec). And it is also clear that Campbell and others perceived the hero from a white, European lens. Many indigenous authors have been critical of how this lens distorted their own stories and traditions. Jan Bourdeau Waboose (Waboose and Deines 2002), an indigenous children's author, Alanis Obomsawin (2017), an indigenous filmmaker, and elders Elizabeth Greenland, Mary Kendi, Annie Norbert, Gabe Andre, and Eunice Mitchell (Kennedy *et al.*, 2009), and others, have told traditional stories, ensuring that the format, structure, and telling are all from the specific indigenous culture's point of view.

The idea of the hero and the hero's journey has many limitations and blind spots in terms of gender, race, culture, sexual orientation, and identity. However, to me, a true mythic journey cannot be a singular archetypal experience. Everyone is different, and will be motivated, inspired, and taught by varying archetypal images and yearnings. The goal is ultimately to discover our own inner voice, and to uncover our own personal hidden stories. If that is our journey, then we may identify with many archetypes along the way, even if they are from a different culture, tradition, or gender; I believe that at the most basic level, Campbell's (2008, 2011, 2017) "hero's journey" is equally applicable to all individuals regardless of gender or sexual identity, culture, race, or sexual orientation. The hero, or protagonist, is not a person, but an archetype, a set of universal images combined with specific patterns of behavior that are useful as a template for working with the *Story Within* with an understanding of the cultural limitations. Interestingly, I have found that Campbell's template not only applies to the stories themselves but also to the personal process of those going through the *Story Within*. Campbell outlines 17 steps in his monomyth, and Christopher Vogler (2007) took this 17-stage monomyth and shaped it into a 12-stage model. In my work the 12-stage model covers all the necessary steps. And while not all 12 steps are present in every mythic story, many of them are, even if just touched on. The personal meaning within an archetypal story does not come from the literal but rather from the metaphors and symbols. In understanding the symbolic meaning of a myth, we come to know the psychological undercurrent—including hidden motivations, tensions, and desires within our own psyche. Battling inner and outer demons, forging ahead on a dangerous path, confronting fears, all of these symbolize our own personal passage through day-to-day life. The mythic and our daily lives are always intertwined and exist simultaneously. This connection between the profound and prosaic is what leads to self-discovery, and transformation.

The following is an outline and brief description of each of the 12 stages based on Campbell's work. I have also included an example from a myth, fairy tale, or traditional story, and a sense of how this stage can be identified in the *Story Within* process.

The 12 Stages of the Hero's Journey, Based on Campbell (2008) and Vogel (2007)

1. Ordinary World

STORY

As with any narrative, before an adventure can begin the hero exists in their ordinary world with specific norms, customs, conditioned beliefs, and behaviors. In the story it is necessary to establish what this ordinary world is, even if brief and fantastical. This is where the journey begins.

Examples:

- Cinderella cleaning and covered in ashes (*Cendrillon*, Perrault)
- Persephone collecting flowers in a field (Persephone, Greek)
- Harry Potter sleeping in a cupboard under the stairs (Harry Potter, Rowling)

THE *STORY WITHIN* PROCESS

What is the current situation and state of mind of the client? Where do they live, with whom, and do they work or go to school? How do they describe their day-to-day environment?

2. Call to Adventure

STORY

The hero's adventure begins when they receive some sort of call to action, such as a direct threat to themselves or their community. It may not be that dramatic, but whatever it is, and however it manifests itself, it ultimately disrupts the comfort of the hero's "ordinary world" and presents a challenge or quest that must be undertaken.

Examples:

- Hansel and Gretel left in the woods ("Hansel and Gretel," Grimm)
- Frodo visited by Gandalf (*The Lord of the Rings*, Tolkien)

- Sedna discovers the man she married is really a bird in disguise (Sedna, Inuit)

The *Story Within* Process

This is the stage when the client begins the *Story Within* journey and commits to the process of creative projection and looking for a story. There is also a call to action—a sense that there is something hidden and inaccessible that is causing discomfort in their life and relationships, and they feel the call to a quest into their own unconscious.

3. Refusal of the Call

Story

Although the hero may be eager to embark on the quest, fear and doubt can often lead them to question their ability to face the challenges ahead. Their ordinary world is so familiar, and the comfort of home far more attractive than the perilous journey into the unknown.

Examples:

- Frodo offers the ring to Gandalf (*The Lord of the Rings*, Tolkien)
- Zaleukos refusing to follow the unknown man ("The Story of the Hewn-off Hand," Arabic)
- Dinoysia, a princess, is chosen by the king to be his wife; she weeps and tries to oppose the marriage, telling her woes to Labismena, the sea serpent ("Why the Sea Moans," Brazilian)

The *Story Within* Process

The search for the "right" story can be an arduous process and bring up feelings of self-doubt, confusion, and not wanting to continue.

4. Meeting with the Mentor, Supernatural Aid, Magical Allies

Story

Initially, the hero can resist change, but ultimately they decide to embark on the adventure. Often this decision occurs when the hero encounters someone or something that offers an encouraging word, gift, or vision that helps in preparation for the journey ahead. Whatever the hero is given, it serves to dispel their doubts and fears and gives them the strength and courage to begin their quest.

Examples:

- Khoai meeting the Buddha in the jungle ("The Hundred-Knot Bamboo," Vietnamese)

- King Arthur meeting Merlin (*King Arthur and His Knights of the Round Table*, Arthurian)

- Red Riding Cap meets the wolf ("Red Riding Cap," Grimm)

The *Story Within* Process
As the client struggles to find and trust their inner sense of "knowing" what the "right" story is, something happens that is unexpected, and appears as a sign to continue. This can be in the form of a dream, an image, a meaningful encounter with someone, or a piece of music, that in some way helps them to make a decision and choose the story.

5. *Crossing the First Threshold*
Story
The hero leaves their ordinary world for the first time and crosses the threshold into adventure. Once the hero steps across the crumbling bridge, starts on an overgrown and winding forest path, or dives into forbidding waters, there is no turning back. The first threshold marks a major decision: they are committed to the quest whether it be physical, spiritual, or emotional, even though they may be afraid. This first breakthrough is important and necessary; however, it is but the first of many turning points.

Examples:

- Goorialla, the rainbow serpent traveling across Australia to find their tribe ("The Rainbow Serpent," Australian, aboriginal)

- Dorothy lifted into the air in the tornado (*The Wonderful Wizard of Oz*, Baum)
- Persephone abducted in Hades (Persephone, Greek)

THE *STORY WITHIN* PROCESS
Once the story and character are chosen, the client starts to engage with their unconscious through different creative mediums. Even though they do not know where the process will lead, they are willing to enter the unknown and accept whatever emerges as part of their journey.

6. Trials and Tribulations
STORY
As the hero moves forward on their journey, they must endure trials and tribulations and painfully learn the rules of this mythic world. Obstacles are thrown across their path, whether they be physical hurdles or demons, monsters, or other humans bent on thwarting their progress. The hero needs to find out who can be trusted and who cannot, and how each enemy and ally is necessary to prepare for the greater ordeals yet to come. This is the stage where skills and/or powers are tested, and every obstacle faced helps the hero to gain a deeper insight and courage.
   Examples:

- Hercules forced to accomplish the ten labors by his enemy Eurystheus (Hercules, Greek)
- Miller's daughter having to spin straw into gold (Rumpelstiltskin, Grimm)
- Ugly duckling having to endure abuse and neglect (Ugly Duckling, Andersen)

THE *STORY WITHIN* PROCESS
Working with diverse creative mediums and their unconscious, clients are faced with the enemies and obstacles of their character and begin to feel their character's discomfort and fear in a deeply personal way.

They may find that aspects of their character's personality start to come through in their own lives in unexpected ways. A challenge faced in real life may mirror the challenge faced by their chosen character.

7. Approaching the Inmost Cave
Story

The inmost cave can be represented by many things in the hero's story such as an actual location which lies hidden and surrounded by danger, a treasure or supernatural being buried or out of reach, or an inner conflict which up until now the hero has not had to face. When the hero approaches the cave, they may discover that whatever they are doing is not working and once again they face doubts and fears that they will not be able to succeed. They may need some time to stop, reflect, and try a different approach. This brief respite helps the hero understand the magnitude of the ordeal that awaits and escalates the tension in anticipation of the ultimate test.

Examples:

- Monkey reflecting after discovering he has dragged home a snarling wild dog ("Papa Bois and Monkey Trouble," Trinidad)

- Gretel planning an escape from the witch's cage ("Hansel and Gretel," Grimm)

- Theseus contemplates how to get through the labyrinth ("Theseus and the Minotaur," Greek)

The *Story Within* Process

As clients begin to come closer to their own hidden story, they often feel stuck as if they are not making progress. This hidden story has been defended for a long time and will not reveal itself easily. The client will need to stop, rest, and ultimately find a new approach to be able to continue this process.

8. Ordeal

STORY

The ordeal may be a dangerous physical test or a deep inner crisis that the hero must face to survive or to protect their community or the world. Whether it be facing their greatest fear or most deadly foe, the hero draws upon all their skills and experiences thus far to overcome this most difficult challenge. Only through some form of "death" can the hero be reborn, experiencing a metaphorical resurrection that gives them the power or insight needed to fulfill their destiny. This is the high point of the hero's journey, where everything is put on the line—life as they know it will never be the same again.

Examples:

- When the grandmother throws Seal Boy into the ocean (Seal Boy, Inuit)
- Aphrodite making Psyche accomplish three tasks to win Eros back (Eros and Psyche, Greek)
- Inanna going through the trials when she enters the land of the dead (Inanna, Sumerian)

THE *STORY WITHIN* PROCESS

The client faces a dangerous internal test which can come in many forms but always involves a crucial turning point. To truly let go of being controlled by a hidden story in the unconscious, the client needs to let the old self die. This ordeal can be terrifying, as the client must shed the skin of the familiar and the known and trust that this shedding and destruction of the old self will lead to something better and more fulfilling. There is a sadness and a mourning that needs to take place before they can continue.

9. Revelation, Transformation

STORY

After defeating the enemy, surviving death, and finally overcoming their greatest personal challenge, the hero is ultimately transformed and rewarded. The reward may come in many forms: in an object of

Elements in Myths, Fairy Tales, and Traditional Stories   89

power or immense importance, a secret revealed, greater knowledge or insight, or even reconciliation with a loved one or ally. Whatever the treasure, the hero must begin the return home.

Examples:

- Angajuk whipped Kautjajuq until he grew into a giant and Shaman (Kautjajuq, Inuit)

- Kroemoe, King of the Crows, pulls Towei up into the blue sky with him and she is transformed into Queen of the Crows (Queen of the Crows, Caribbean)

- Ugly duckling realizes that it is really a swan (Ugly Duckling, Andersen)

THE *STORY WITHIN* PROCESS
After the old self dies there is a sense of relief and rebirth and the client feels as if they have found what they were looking for. The connection between the story and character and their own lives becomes clear and insight occurs naturally.

10. *The Road Back*
STORY
The hero begins their journey back to their ordinary life. They look forward to returning with their new-found treasure and wisdom. But the hero's journey is not yet over, and they may still need one last push back into the "ordinary world." The moment before the hero finally commits to the last stage of their journey may be a moment in which they must choose between their own personal objective and that of a higher cause.

Examples:

- Hi'iaku agrees to retrieve the dead Lohi'au, and on the journey back Lohi'au is killed and dies again but is then resurrected (Pele, Goddess of Fire, Hawaiian)

- Harry willingly sacrifices himself to Voldemort, and appears dead but is not (Harry Potter, Rowling)

- Beauty goes back to be with the dying beast ("Beauty and the Beast," Lang)

The *Story Within* Process
After making important story/character life connections, the client is ready to return to their old life but with new insights and new possibilities. They look forward to sharing their insights but are unsure how they will integrate their new wisdom into their ordinary life.

11. Death and Resurrection
Story
The hero faces an unexpected and final test where they have a dangerous encounter with death. Everything is at stake because if they fail it will have far-reaching consequences not only for the hero but also for their ordinary world and the lives of those left behind. Ultimately the hero will succeed and emerge from battle cleansed and reborn.

Examples:

- Zeulokos is identified as a murderer and sentenced to death. An old friend, Valetty, emerges, to try and save his life ("The Story of the Hewn-off Hand," Arabic)

- Outa Karel unknowingly calls to Death to find him, bids the *baasjes* adieu for the night, promises to tell another story the next day, and lives to tell many great stories ("The Ostrich Hunt," South African)

- Inanna is killed by Ereshkigal in the underworld but then resurrected (Inanna, Sumerian)

The *Story Within* Process
On their way back to their ordinary life, clients are faced with the ultimate challenge of confronting their deepest fear of change. They have now uncovered their hidden story and understand how this story has affected their lives. They have an opportunity to return to their family and friends as a different person with new insights and ways

of responding and engaging. However, they are faced with death—the old self and habits must die. This can be terrifying and will call upon all the inner strength they have gained in the journey.

12. Return with Elixir
STORY
This is the final stage where the hero brings their knowledge or the "elixir" back into the ordinary world. The elixir may be many things either metaphoric or literal. It could be a cause for celebration, self-realization, or an end to strife, but it represents change, and proof that the hero left the ordinary world and returned as a different person. They will have grown, confronted many dangers, even death, and now look forward to sharing their wisdom with others.

Examples:

- Jack coming back with the treasure ("Jack and the Beanstalk," Jacobs)

- Dorothy coming back home with new realizations (*The Wonderful Wizard of Oz*, Baum)

- Tailfeather Woman instructs her people to make a ceremonial drum (Tailfeather Woman, Ojibwe)

THE *STORY WITHIN* PROCESS
Clients have found a way to communicate their transformation through a creative medium and are willing to share this with others. They have returned to their ordinary world with wisdom and insight and are able to integrate the new learning into their interpersonal interactions with both their outer and inner worlds.

Key Archetypal Themes, Based on da Silva (2017) and Others

In addition to the stages of the hero's journey, there also some key archetypal themes that are often present in myths, fairy tales, and traditional stories.

Resurrection

This theme is related to rebirth and a return to life after death. It is often connected to spring and the finalizing of a cycle. Death is seen as a metaphor, not only as pain and loss but also as the possibility of rebirth. From a psychological perspective, death and resurrection is when all the parts of the self are recognized and integrated.

Examples:

- Ademis: reborn as a flower (Babylonian, Greek)
- Buddha: reincarnation (Indian, Chinese, Japanese)
- Bear Man: killed by tribe, then resurrected (Cherokee)

Miraculous Birth and Dangers from the Environment

This theme is related to the origins and initial environment of the protagonist of the story. A recurrent motif is the idea of something miraculous or unusual about the birth itself and something dangerous about the environment.

Examples:

- Perseus. Miraculous birth: son of Zeus and a mortal woman. Danger: mother and child locked in a wooden chest in the sea washed ashore and saved by fisherman (Perseus, Greek)
- Queen of Assyria. Miraculous birth: the half-mortal daughter of a fish goddess is abandoned in the wilderness, fed by doves, survives, and becomes Semiramis, the great Warrior Queen of Assyria. Danger: fish goddess who abandons her to die (Warrior Queen of Assyria, Assyrian)
- Remus and Romulus. Miraculous birth: the twins are left exposed on the banks of the Tiber and are suckled and fed by a wolf and a woodpecker and survive. Danger: King Amulius who orders them to die (Remus and Romulus, Roman)

Childhood: Fighting Monsters and Meeting the Divine

This theme is related to the direct interactions between the protagonist and monsters or demons and with a divine or supernatural being.

Often the hero must contend with an obstacle that they must overcome and at the same time they meet an ally who has the power to help.
Examples:

- Jack has divine intervention when the beans turn into a giant beanstalk and then fights the giant ("Jack and the Beanstalk," Jacobs)
- Dionysus, captured by pirates, is saved by turning into a lion (Dionysus, Greek)
- Cinderella is abused by her stepmother and stepsisters before divine intervention from her Fairy Godmother or tree at her mother's grave (*Cendrillon*, Perrault)

Meditation, Withdrawal, Reflection

This theme relates to the idea that for the hero to succeed they need to stop, reflect, and separate from the world. This withdrawal is necessary to be able to receive wisdom, fight the dragon, approach the enemy, or find the treasure.
Examples:

- Buddha meditates under a tree (Buddhist texts)
- Percival the Knight withdraws to castle to be educated by mentor (*King Arthur and His Knights of the Round Table*, Arthurian)
- La Loba: Wolf Woman retreats to her cave to sing over the bones (La Loba, Pueblo)

Quest

This theme is crucial to most archetypal stories where the hero must embark on an adventure or quest. The goal of the quest can vary greatly from rescuing a family member, recovering a lost treasure, gaining wisdom and insight, to saving the community from disaster, and the list goes on.
Examples:

- Frodo must destroy the ring (*The Lord of the Rings*, Tolkien)
- Theseus seeks the minotaur and goes into the labyrinth ("Theseus and the Minotaur," Greek)
- Demeter goes in search of her daughter Persephone (Demeter and Persephone, Greek)
- Orpheus goes in search of Eurydice (Orpheus and Eurydice, Greek)

Descent

In many stories the hero descends into an underworld. While there, they are faced with death, terror, demons, and ultimately the potential for rebirth and transformation.

Examples:

- Inanna/Ishtar, descent into underworld (Babylonian, Sumerian)
- Persephone's descent into Hades (Greek)
- Orpheus' descent into Hades to retrieve Eurydice (Orpheus and Eurydice, Greek)
- Quan Yin, Goddess of Mercy, had the opportunity to ascend to paradise but chose to descend to Earth to alleviate suffering (Chinese, Buddhist)
- Emperor Yudhishthira got to heaven but then descended to one of the underworlds to find his brothers (*Mahabharata*, Hindu)

Trickster/Shapeshifter

In many cultures there is a character (god, goddess, spirit, man, woman, animal) who often exhibits gender and form fluidity, has a cunning intellect, and disobeys normal rules and conventional behavior. The trickster, or shapeshifter, likes to cause mischief and play tricks but can also be the one to save the community or the hero from harm.

Examples:

- Loki shape-shifted into a mare and became impregnated by a stallion, creating the race of eight-legged horses called Sleipnir; Freyja, the goddess of love and fertility, had a cloak of feather falcons which allowed her to transform into a falcon at will; likewise, Odin was fond of transforming into the shape of an eagle (Norse)

- Selkies, a type of seal that could turn into a human, played in the ocean, while the kelpie, a water spirit that could turn into a horse or woman, dwelled in the lakes and rivers (Celtic)

- An evil fairy cast a spell turning a prince into a beast ("Beauty and the Beast," Lang)

- Coyote as a trickster is hailed as a hero for helping humans by stealing fire and killing monsters (Navaho)

- Iktomi, a shapeshifter spider spirit, can take any shape including that of a human and is seen as both good and bad (Lakota Sioux)

The stages of the hero's journey and the archetypal themes are meant to be guidelines and touchstones with which to assess whether a story fits into a mythic framework. Most myths, fairy tales, and traditional stories will have at least some of these elements and therefore will work well for the *Story Within* process. As you look through the examples for each stage of the hero's journey and for the key archetypal themes, you may be inspired to search out some of these stories and be led to the very one that is waiting for you to find it…

CHAPTER 7

How to Go Through the Steps

It is now time to enter the process. The order of the steps have been carefully thought out and I recommend you do them in sequence. Each step is designed to safely guide you through an inner journey using all the creative mediums and an existing myth, fairy tale, or traditional story to discover your own hidden inner story. The steps are meant to be followed in your own time and in your own way. However, there are some specific guidelines that are necessary to help you prepare and set up your space, get equipment, and find your circle of support.

> I strongly recommend you do this process within the context of a group. However, if this is not feasible, it can be done individually with another professional in the context of your personal therapy. In this case your therapist would be the witness and engage in the creative work with you. Since I have designed the steps in each exercise to be in the context of a group, please modify accordingly. Clinically, I have found the process to be effective with both groups and individuals.

Circle of Support

As mentioned above, before you enter the process of the *Story Within*, you need to set up a strong container to ensure that you are safe. It is essential to have someone else there to be a witness and to work with you in several of the creative exercises. If it is feasible, I strongly encourage you to have a circle of support made up of other therapists, or professionals, who have a strong interest in self-reflection and engaging in a personal journey. If this is not feasible, or you are concerned about what might emerge, you can do this process as part of your own personal therapy. It is best if all of the members of this circle are going through the *Story Within* at the same time. This way you can support each other throughout the process and ensure that all members are safe (for specific details about this, please see the witnessing section in Chapter 5, "Therapeutic Frame").

Circle of Support Guidelines

1. This book is geared towards clinicians, therapists, creative arts therapists, and community workers. As with any deep personal process, difficult material can arise. If you, or anyone else in your circle, are fragile, suicidal, or are concerned in any way about what might emerge in this process, please seek another professional for help. This book cannot take the place of therapy. It is important that everyone in your circle is stable enough to go through a deep internal process.

2. It is most helpful if everyone in your group goes through the *Story Within* process and follows the sequence together. This way you can witness each other and work creatively together for several exercises.

3. Throughout the book I will provide the steps of the creative exercises and it may be helpful to do these creative steps while in the presence of your witnesses. This could mean that you all do your personal creations and explorations at the same time in the same room and then come together to share. Or you take turns being the witness for each other's creative process. Either way will work, but you should establish a structure and follow it throughout the process.

4. Establish a set time, day, and duration for your witnessing (once a week on the same day and time for at least two hours is best).

5. Agree to a verbal or written contract to establish how you will give feedback, maintain confidentiality, and let each other know if you have concerns about the other person's safety.

6. Take a non-interpretative and non-judgmental stance (please see Chapter 5, "Therapeutic Frame," for more details). In order to allow for each person to be safe and to truly experience their own process, it is essential that other members of the group (or friends, family, etc.) do not interpret, or give advice about, what comes up. If you give your interpretation for someone else, it robs them of their own discovery and process. Feedback should be supportive and cover what moved you personally but should not be an interpretation of what has come up for someone else.

Supplies

You need to get some basic creative supplies that will allow you to explore your creativity with different mediums. They do not have to be elaborate, but you need to ensure that you have some basic materials. If money is an issue, you can find many supplies in the dollar store, get donations from art supply stores or schools, and can use recycled materials. If you work with a circle of support, you can buy materials together and in bulk. It doesn't matter at all if you have the most extensive supplies or just a few basic ones. What matters is that you have a few items from each medium (art, music, drama/dance, writing). Below are some recommendations for each modality, but please only purchase what fits into your budget and space limitations.

Art

Paint (water color, acrylic), different sized paint brushes, containers for water, pastels (chalk, oil), permanent markers, crayons, colored pencils, different sizes and textures of paper, clay, glue, glue gun, needles and thread, charcoal, stapler, masking tape, rubber bands, glitter, marbles, feathers, cotton balls, ribbons, boxes of different sizes, recycled containers of all sizes and shapes, blank masks, hockey helmets, baseball gloves, found objects, bark, moss, nails, shells, rocks, etc. (Go to stores, look on the streets, see what you have, and enjoy!)

Music
A few percussion instruments (small drums, shakers, blocks, and you can also use pots and pans). Wooden paddles to use with percussion (works well on pots and pans), any instruments you already play and have, recorders, kalimba, xylophone, triangles, chimes, bells, and of course your voice!

Drama/Dance

- Fabric: Sheets, blankets, scarves, bedspreads; you can go to a fabric store and pick out different materials, colors, and textures.

- Props: Rope, wire, nails, straw, boxes, fake swords, flowers, chains, small rugs, fairy lights (basically anything that can be used as a prop to create a scene or an environment).

- Costumes: Old hats, dresses, pants, goggles, Halloween costumes, feather boas, scarves (anything that can be used as a costume for your character).

Writing
A journal. It can be a notebook you have lying around, your computer or iPad, even your phone. The important aspect is that it needs to be a consistent place where you document your journey. Pencils, pens, markers, etc. for writing titles and text on art work.

The Studio
To create you need to have a designated space where you can feel free to move, get messy, and make noise. It does not have to be anything fancy, or expensive, or large, just an area where you can keep some creative supplies. Sometimes you can find a community space where you can have a locker for storage, or a basement in someone's house

who is willing to be the "host" for a group of people going through the process. The important aspect is that it is a consistent space that you use to go through the steps of the *Story Within*.

The fun part (budget permitting) is to go to thrift stores, dollar stores, and art, musical, and fabric stores and explore what you are drawn to. This will initiate the process of developing and listening to your own intuition.

Not Knowing

It can be a challenge to stay with "not knowing" and refrain from interpreting and analysis. The thing is, we will interpret, and we will analyze. However, we can recognize this in ourselves and learn to let interpretations and analyses go, just as we would in meditation when thoughts come and go. We can see the interpretations and analyses like leaves on a river; they are present, floating along, and we watch them float by without holding on to them or creating a narrative about them. Not easy to do, but ultimately the more we can trust and rest in "not knowing," the more we can truly be led to discover something new and access a hidden aspect of ourselves.

Ritual for Entering and Exiting the Process

To stay safe and to honor each step it is important to develop your own rituals for entering and exiting the process. For example, designate a specific space that will be your creative space throughout the process. And find a way that you will call your character and enter your character and do the same for when you de-role or leave your character. This is essential for ensuring safety.

Objects and Documentation

Objects can become especially important throughout this process and it is important to find a way to contain the objects (masks, costumes, etc.) in boxes, fabric, closets, etc. You will need to make these decisions as you go along. It is essential that you document your process in photographs, writing, audio recordings, etc. so that at the very end you can look over the entire process from beginning to end. Keep a journal!

Attitude

- Have compassion for yourself and others.
- There is no "right" way to create. Whatever feels authentic and true for you is your guide.
- Let go of judgment—or at least learn to recognize and laugh with your inner critic.
- Embrace discomfort—consider it necessary for growth.
- Celebrate imperfection.
- Stay safe—listen to your own warning signs, and if you feel unsafe, stop and seek help.
- Be open to discovery—this is an adventure into the realms of your inner world.
- Observe patterns in symbols, metaphors, colors, textures, sounds, and movements.
- Develop *Open Attention* (a state of listening quietly without expectations or effort, an inner stillness and silence so that the mind can rest in "simple presence").
- Develop *Direct Intention*—a state of focussed concentration on a specific creative task, immersing yourself in the medium, not being distracted by thoughts or environment).
- Let go of interpretation and having an agenda.
- Enter the unknown.
- Be open to your own creative DNA and explore the different mediums.

- Take all the time you need for each step—it is fine to spend weeks on Step 1 if that feels right.
- Learn to listen to your deepest inner voice, your intuition, and your own personal sense of "knowing."
- Let yourself have fun and play.
- Develop a ritual for entering and exiting each step of the process.
- Allow yourself to be held and supported by your witnesses.
- Be a holding and supportive witness.
- Be wild, be still, be silly, be heartbroken, be whatever comes through at each step.

To help with safety, please go through the process in the order presented. Each step prepares you for the next step and the one after that. From my experience in creating and working with this process for over 20 years, to be able to access parts of ourselves that have remained hidden we need to go slowly and trust that the arts, and the character we choose, will lead us where we need to go…

I wish you a wonderful adventure…

> My basement studio is a mess. Art supplies scattered on the floor, musical instruments left unplayed, a wooden floor not danced on… For too many years I have abandoned my creativity, accepted that my university job was more important and pressing. Today, looking out on a bright winter day with snow blowing in a chilling wind, I begin this process of rediscovery; I decide that my creativity cannot wait any longer…and slowly I enter my studio and breathe deeply…

Part II

STEPS OF THE PROCESS

CHAPTER 8

Encounter

She entered the room full of shame, her eyes looking down, her body hunched. She spoke in a whisper… At ten years old she carried the weight of the world on her shoulders. Sadly, she suffered horrible pain from Crohn's disease and had a colostomy bag. She told me that her parents felt she had this disease because they were not religious enough. She sat down and prepared herself for a discussion about pain management and self-esteem. Instead I pointed to the objects in the center of the room and told her we would be going on a creative journey. I asked her to encounter the objects as if she was an alien from space and had no idea what they were. She giggled and began the process. I invited her to use different creative mediums to express her own reaction to the objects. She began building with clay, then moved on to a very tentative movement and ended with a song. Then she looked at me with bright eyes and asked, "Is this really therapy—it was so much fun!" I smiled and we looked over her creations. I asked her to teach me the song and she did. She left the room humming the song and smiling…the hospital doctors and nurses asked why she looked happy and I said she had an "encounter"…

When we truly engage in a creative process we become totally absorbed, our senses come alive, and the rest of the world falls away. We see something, really see it, as if for the first time. It calls to us, seduces us, so that we must pay attention and respond. The response comes through us as a poem, a song, a dance… According to Rollo May (1994) this heightened state of consciousness is an encounter, or what he calls genuine creativity. Once we have a true encounter with something it becomes personal and is imbued with meaning.

As Martin Buber (1937, 2004) tells us, having an "I–thou" relationship is different from an "I–it" relationship. When we experience the "I–thou" there is an intimacy and we are participants addressing another as a presence. The same intimacy can happen when we begin the process of creative projection (described in detail in Chapter 2). Some object, idea, feeling, or scene calls out to us. And if we follow the call then we feel compelled to respond through a personal creative expression. I believe this creative call and response is within our DNA and comes naturally. All we need to do is extend an invitation.

As a child, responding to life creatively was as natural as breathing. We all engaged in play and pretend as a part of the learning process. The ability to playfully explore the world within as well as our environment is often lost as we age into adulthood. It becomes repressed as we feel we must conform to many societal and cultural pressures. As we begin the *Story Within* process, we are reconnecting with our inherent creativity and our childhood. For some of us there are childhood memories that are difficult and painful, yet even within this there are the memories of playful abandon. One of the pleasures of working creatively is that we reclaim our inherent joyful creativity. As we create, we bring something new into being, something that did not exist before we produced it. It is our unique voice and expression. To be creative we must live in ambiguity and yet have complete conviction. We are open to the unexpected and the exploration of the unknown and yet at the same time we are focussed on our medium and the specific materials and form to express what we need to. It is this paradox of existing in both the known and the unknown, the free abandon and the focussed attention, that allows for what May (1994) calls genuine creativity.

Stages of Encounter (According to Rollo May 1994)

1. *Seeing*. Seeing an object as if for the first time. Something stands out, seduces us, captures our attention. It can be an internal or external focus, for example one tree in a forest, or one idea.

2. *Absorption.* Direct focus, not distracted by anything, fully absorbed by an object or idea rather than the self.

3. *Response.* Personal response to an object with emotional and cognitive engagement, relationship with an object imbued with personal words, feelings, and images.

4. *Sensory.* Heightened awareness with all the senses engaged.

5. *New Paradigm.* Bringing something new into being, something that has never been there before, that is our unique creation.

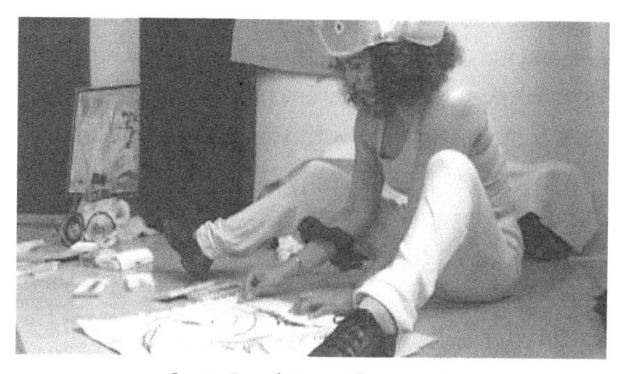

Sonja Boodajee with artwork

Relationship to Creativity

Before we begin the *Story Within* process it is important to get a sense of our relationship to our own creativity. To do this, here are the steps to follow (you can do this alone or with your circle of support):

1. Write down three words that come to mind quickly when you think of creativity (allow no more than one to two minutes for this).

2. How close to your body do you feel your creativity is right now (far away in another room, inside your belly, on the tips of your fingers…)? Indicate this physically.

3. Where in your body do you feel your creativity (hands, breath, head)?

Make sure to write all your responses in your journal. It will be interesting to review it once you have completed the *Story Within* process. Share your responses with your circle of support.

THE ENCOUNTER EXERCISE

To begin the *Story Within* process we begin with an exercise I call *The Encounter*. An archetypal object (or objects) is placed in the middle of the room and everyone is asked to encounter it and then respond creatively to the object through all the different mediums. This exercise is necessary to give a direct experience of creative projection in a safe and distanced way. Clients are introduced to all the mediums with a sense of curiosity, non-judgment, and fun. Doing all the different mediums is essential because it exposes us right away to the different mediums and establishes a sense of inquiry as to our relationship with the mediums. It also allows us to witness our own creative process without judgment. There is no right or wrong way to do the creative expression.

Preparation
Object to Encounter
You need to set up an archetypal object in the middle of the room. I use three ornate golden small goblets on a red gossamer scarf. The scarf is draped over a stool and the three goblets are placed in a circle in the middle of the stool. These objects work in a Western context and can elicit a sense of the mythic or archetypal. They are both prosaic and profound and not too specific or limiting. The objects will be different for each culture, and what is considered archetypal will also differ depending on the cultural symbols and stories. For example, for some Asian cultures there could be the Yin/Yang symbol, a rice bowl, or teacup, and indigenous cultures might have an animal skin, a drum, or a feather. Each culture will have different symbols that elicit an archetypal sense of meaning. The goal is to have it be both familiar and yet also mysterious, so it can be inviting and conducive to a creative response.

Creative Mediums (whatever budget will permit)

- Art: Varied sizes, colors, textures, of paper, pastels, paints, brushes, clay, charcoal, yarn, feathers, glitter, twigs, shells, rocks, nails, moss, wire, glue, scissors, glue gun, stapler. Any material can be used in art: recyclable egg containers, plastic, etc. Fabric: scarves, sheets, assorted colors and textures from fabric store, ribbon, yarn.

- Music: Percussion instruments: blocks, small drums, pots and pans, shakers, rain stick, kalimba, bells; any other instruments you have (recorder, guitar, piano, etc.). You can use art materials for sound (shaking paper, snapping scissors, paintbrush against glass—be creative!).

- Journal to write in.

Please remember to try and have fun and not judge yourself. It is perfectly fine if you have no experience with any of the creative mediums, just explore them as if you were a child or an alien from another planet. The goal of this exercise is to become familiar with the different mediums and with the idea of creative projection. It also brings home how unique we all are and that each of our creative responses will be different.

The Encounter

1. Place an archetypal object (or objects) in the center of the room.

2. Look at it from many angles: up, down, beneath, far away, close.

3. *Encounter* some aspect of the object that you are drawn to (could be the inside of one goblet, the scarf, or even the space under the stool). It does not matter what it is and there is no right and wrong; just pay attention to what calls you.

4. Do a creative response with different mediums. Do the following in any order you wish but you must do *all* the mediums:

    i. Make an *artistic creation* (draw, paint, sculpt with clay, shape fabrics on the floor, make a collage, etc.).

ii. *Embody* the object through a postural shape and movement.

iii. Make a *sound* that expresses the object (with instruments, paper, or other objects, voice, etc.).

iv. *Write* a first-person story from the perspective of the object, beginning with "I am the…" (with a limit of one page).

5. After you have done all the mediums, give your artistic creation a title and put the title either on the artistic piece or beside it.

6. Give your story a title. Look over your story and choose four lines that express the essence of your story. Highlight or circle these four lines.

7. Reflection: In your journal answer the following questions:

   i. What was the order of the mediums? Which one did you do first, second, etc.?

   ii. Which medium did you spend the most time with?

   iii. Which medium did you spend the least time with?

   iv. Which medium was most comfortable?

   v. Which medium was least comfortable?

   vi. Which medium was the most emotional or touched you the most?

   vii. Which medium touched you the least?

   viii. Which medium was the most fun?

   ix. Which medium do you wish you had spent more time with?

8. In looking over all your answers, does anything surprise you? If so, what? The above reflections can begin to reveal your creative DNA. You may be surprised by your experience of the different mediums and by your reflections. Stay honest and open and see what emerges…

9. Either meet in partners or in your circle of support and share whatever creations you wish to share. Witnesses should be supportive, holding space, and can ask questions and share their own personal response. The questions and personal response are all in service of the other person and are not an interpretation or analysis.

Working with Clients

I use three archetypal golden goblets and a red scarf draped over a stool. You need to choose what is appropriate for the culture(s) you are working with. I find that archetypal objects work best to elicit deeper and less specific responses. This is an essential first step and can serve as an assessment tool. Can the client make a creative projection? Does it work for them on some level, through at least one of the mediums? Witnessing the client engaging with all the mediums gives you a sense of their creative DNA from your observations and from their own personal reflection. The process is a mutual discovery. The language of creativity becomes central and forms a bridge between you and your client, a communication that is both intimate and safe. There is no confrontation, no interpretation, just a sense of beginning a journey together.

In this exercise there is one communal object that creates a sense of being part of a group and yet at the same time being internally focussed. The directive of having to engage with all the mediums is essential because it exposes the client right away to the different mediums and establishes a sense of inquiry as to their personal relationship with the mediums. Which one did they do first or last, and how did each medium affect them? Being forced to work with unfamiliar mediums can take clients out of their comfort zone and allow more unconscious material to come through. As clients become aware of their own judgment, inner critic, desire for perfection, etc., they are developing a sense of an internal witness. It is important to make sure the framework is always about letting go of judgment, embracing imperfection, and maintaining a sense of openness and discovery. This exercise is an important first step in terms of learning a way of self-reflection with the focus on creative process and immediate response rather than interpretation and analysis. As clients share their creative expressions with each other or with you, it becomes clear that every act of creation is unique, and that creative projection can happen quickly and organically and is a direct avenue into the unconscious.

Things to Watch Out For

- *Too many materials in the room can feel overwhelming.* You need to stand with the clients and introduce them to one or two materials at a time slowly and gradually. Help them choose one or two materials and begin to work with them.

- *Clients refuse to engage with one or all the mediums.* Physically introduce mediums one by one and either sit by them as they explore, or explore the same medium in a quiet way beside them in "mirror play."

- *Clients become overly emotional in one medium.* Help them to find more distance in engaging with another medium or they can direct you to engage with that medium so that they are the director but are not directly working with that medium.

- *A client rushes through all the mediums.* Encourage them to play with the element of time. What would it be like to stay with each medium longer? Ask them to notice if spending more time elicits discomfort and ask them to stay with that medium for a little longer and then notice what happens.

Homework

Let yourself have an encounter. Either inside or outside: set up a period of time where you will allow yourself to be open to what calls you. You will enter an open state, a state of not knowing, of no direction, just open awareness. And whatever calls you, whatever you are drawn to, whether it is a chair, a stop sign, a ray of light coming through the window, or a cat, stop and pay attention and then take a moment for a quick creative response. It can be a poem in your head, a photo on your phone, a movement, or a line from a song. There is no judgment, no right or wrong way of doing this; the only requirement is that you allow yourself to have a creative encounter.

My Process (using three golden goblets and a red scarf draped over a stool)

> I am also going through the *Story Within* steps and will share brief writings from my process. They are just my personal offerings as a part of a large circle of support that includes all of us. Please ignore if distracting.

Four lines that express the essence of my first-person story:

I am the light.

The part of the goblet that sings, that dances, that seeks God.

Sometimes I have trouble seeing myself and
  get lost in the darkness around me.

Does the light ever die?

CHAPTER 9

Chaos and Order

I entered the room and saw a skeletally thin girl sitting up in bed hooked up to a heart monitor. I introduced myself and sat at the edge of her bed. She was admitted to the hospital because she had severe anorexia and her heart was affected. She was 16 but looked around 11. I felt something squishy under the covers and found, to my dismay, old uneaten food hidden there. She started to deny that it was hers, but without saying a word I wrapped the food in Kleenex and threw it out. And then I surprised her by asking if she liked fairy tales. Immediately her face changed into a big smile and she said she loved "The Wizard of Oz." For several months we worked together with this story. She refused all other forms of therapy and continued to be non-compliant about re-feeding but agreed to see me because I never spoke about eating or her weight. Instead, within the limitations of her hospital bed, she made masks, costumes, art work, and embodied characters from the Wizard of Oz. She identified as Dorothy and told me that the tornado was "good" because it took her to the sacred place of Oz, where she felt special and in control, whereas Good Witch Glenda was "evil" and tried to get her to betray the tornado and send her back to Kansas. To feel a sense of "order" in her life she had to abstain from eating (the tornado) so she could enter the magical world of Oz where she experienced the euphoria of starvation. In contrast, any attempt by the hospital staff to get her to eat was perceived as a direct threat and pushed her directly into "chaos." As time went on, she became thinner and thinner and we were all concerned that her heart would give out and she would die. I understood that until she had a direct experience of the danger of her eating disorder she would not respond to treatment. Instead of challenging her perceptions, I worked with them within the story. I had her embody the tornado and speak as the tornado to her character Dorothy. One day, as she was embodying the tornado, she laughed a maniacal laugh and then came out of role, crying and shivering. For the first time, she experienced the tornado (her anorexia) as malicious and chaotic. This was the start of her recovery. It was a difficult journey, but by working with this story she was able to face her eating disorder and leave the hospital and continue in high school. During a six-month follow-up visit she told me, "I felt so magical in Oz, it provided me a rigid sense of order. I didn't want to return to Kansas and the 'chaos' of eating and feeling myself in my body…it was hard to find out who I was without anorexia. I felt like no one, nothing, so boring in flat Kansas. But now I know the truth about Oz and that the tornado/starvation was not my friend but leading me to death."

The word "chaos" is borrowed from the ancient Greek *Khaos*, meaning void or abyss. This *Khaos* was perceived to be the emptiness or void from which all things evolved and later it became more specific to refer to the abyss of the underworld. In ancient Greek mythology, *Khaos* is depicted as a primordial deity which preceded the order of the cosmos. However, there was a continuous cycle of transformation from "*Khaos*" to "Order." Both are transitory, one leading into the other (Cambridge University Press, 2019). The word "order" is thought to originate from the Latin (*Ordinem*, eleventh century) meaning row, line, rank, pattern, arrangement, routine, "a row of threads in a loom." And as well from the Old French (*Ordre*, thirteenth century) describing those living under a religious discipline, or position, regulation, or rule (Cambridge University Press, 2019). The two words bring together several different cultures and each word carries a sense of both the collective and the personal. For the *Story Within* process it is not so much about the concept of each word but rather the way each concept is personally experienced. We all have a unique internal sense of what chaos and order mean in our own lives, even if we are not aware of it. My internal sense of order may be meditation, yoga, nature, and being by the ocean. Whereas for someone else their internal sense of the same word brings up rigidity, prison, wearing something too tight, being forced into a straight line, and not being able to breathe. Both these responses are valid and there is no one way to experience chaos or order. Rather, it is the process of discovering how these concepts live within each one of us that is important. What makes something chaotic for one person doesn't even register for another, and so we all live within our own framework and often bump against each other in awkward or hostile ways. My chaos could be your order. Essentially, of course, we need both chaos and order to be complete: to merge Apollo, god of light, order, and reason, with Dionysus, god of letting go, chaos, and urging vitality. If there is too much order it can become fanatic and totalitarian; too much chaos can become madness. One is not better than the other; there is no judgment or hierarchy. Ultimately, we want to be able to celebrate our chaos and our order. To do this we need to explore with depth and curiosity how each one lives inside us.

"Invention, it must be humbly admitted, does not consist in creating out of void but out of chaos."

Mary Shelley (1797–1851)

CHAOS AND ORDER EXERCISE

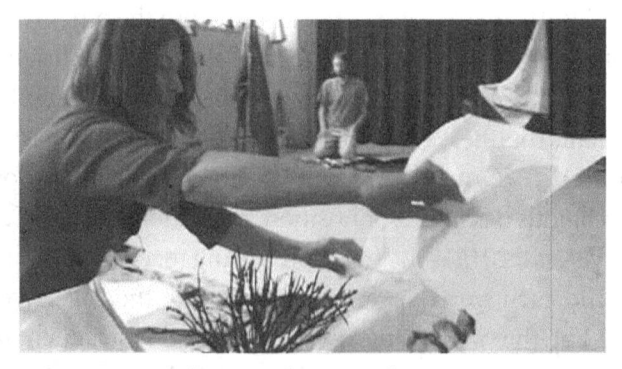

Benedicte Deschamps with creation

Preparation
Space
You need to have space to make two separate creations and also to move.

Materials

The artistic creations for "chaos" and "order" can be made with and on chairs, tables, and furniture using fabric, objects from nature, scarves, costumes, art materials, or things you have lying around. Use your imagination but know that "art" does not have to mean paint on paper; a creation can be putting together strange objects in some sort of form that expresses what each concept means for you.

The Exercise

1. Make two creations that exist separately from each other and from you (not using your own body). Use objects found in the room, in your house, and in nature, and as well you can use your art materials. One creation expresses your feeling of order, and the other creation expresses your feeling of chaos. Please don't think too much and let your intuition and body guide you to the materials that feel right. Start with whichever concept you choose.

2. Once you have completed a creation for chaos and a creation for order, decide on a title for each one and put the title somewhere on or near the creation.

3. Once both creations and title are complete, spend time looking over each one, noticing the colors, shapes, textures, words. Do a quick response to each one using any medium you choose. It could be a poem, a song, a movement, a sketch. It is not important which medium you choose but rather that you do a creative response to each one.

4. Decide how close you feel to each creation. Actually move your body physically towards each one and determine the physical distance that feels right and the position in relationship to the creation. For example, perhaps you feel very close to chaos and lie down on it or feel very distant and place yourself far away, not facing it. Or maybe you are an arm's length from order but facing away. Play with this and explore until you find what feels right.

5. Stand up in front of each creation, and using materials, or not, express order and chaos through embodiment. Find a movement phrase that feels right and a word phrase and/or sound. Be able to repeat your movement, sound, and word phrase over and over, so make sure to be specific.

6. If you are working alone, skip the next exercise, but hopefully you can find someone to do this with (therapist or friend).

7. If you are working in a group, find a partner. Teach your partner your movement/sound/word phrase for order. Then your partner will show it to you, and you correct (gently) anything that isn't right. The goal is for you to be able to witness your own movement and words and to feel free to gently ask for the quality, emotion, expression, and voice you want. Once your partner has the correct embodiment, ask them what they felt like doing this embodiment (no interpretation or judgment, just their own personal experience). Then teach them your movement/sound/word phrase for chaos and go through the same process. Then switch and you now embody your partner's movement/sound/word phrase for chaos and for order. The goal is that you each get to embody someone else's movement/sound/word phrases and witness your own movement/sound/word phrases on someone else. This can be a powerful exercise.

8. Take a photo of your creations. If you want, you can video your partner doing the movement. Or your partner can video you doing your own embodiment.

9. Write about the process in your journal. Which one did you do first: chaos or order? Was one easier to create than the other? Did any feelings or emotions come up when you created order or chaos? If so, what were they and when did they emerge? In looking over your creations, notice any similarities or differences between your chaos and order in terms of colors, shapes, objects, textures, etc. When you look at each one, what are the feelings that come up? Do you enjoy looking at one more than the other? Did anything come up that was surprising?

Working with Clients

Chaos and order are different for each person. The line when something becomes chaos or order is unique and individual. It is important to recognize this in those you work with. You as a therapist also need to know how chaos and order live within you to prevent imposing your experience onto your client. This exercise is also an assessment tool establishing a baseline for what chaos and order mean for your clients. Having a sense of this is an important therapeutic tool so that when their work becomes too chaotic you can remind them of what gives them a sense of order and vice versa. This exercise sets up the idea that there is a duality in all of us and the distinctions between chaos and order are unique to everyone. This also lays a foundation that will emerge throughout the rest of the work.

Things to Watch Out For

- *Clients are not able to express chaos or order or both.* Work with them closely, exploring a variety of materials, asking them what they are drawn to and building the structure with them under their guidance. This will help them feel safe.

- *Clients become overwhelmed with one of their creations, eliciting traumatic memories.* Help them to stop and take distance from their creation and work on the other one (if that is easier for them) and ask them what would help to keep the creation safe. Would they like to put their creation in a box, under a table, or covered in a blanket, so that it is hidden from sight? If it becomes too overwhelming, they should stop. However, if they can continue in a safe way, it may be a crucial step in finding ways to stay safe with difficult feelings.

Homework

- Notice how chaos and order play out in your daily life.
- When do you feel a sense of order, doing what activity?

- When do you feel a sense of chaos?
- Are both enjoyable, or is one uncomfortable?
- What people and relationships feel chaotic or ordered?
- Do some relationships lead you to sing and dance while others feel calming or soothing?
- Notice how and when you transition from chaos to order or order to chaos.

My Process
Chaos

Don't want to look at you
Too raw
Uncovered,
Exposed
Fake Christmas flowers over ski goggles
Nothing fits together and yet,
it does form a whole…

Order

So much space and openness…
yet so grounded
held by the earth (rocks and pinecones)
simple,
not cluttered,
feels so soothing and gentle
I long to be in the center…

CHAPTER 10

Finding and Telling the Story

Sarah was one of a group of students in the class training to be a creative arts therapist. She was intelligent and highly competent. She was also the child of Holocaust survivors. Her parents never spoke about their wartime experience. Instead of a family legacy, there was silence. Sarah suffered from persistent nightmares and unexplained fears. She struggled for a long time, searching through many myths and fairy tales to find the right one to work with. One day, someone told her about the Greek myth of Pandora's Box and she immediately knew this was her story. Pandora was given a box and told that the box contained special gifts, but she was not allowed to ever open the box. Eventually Pandora's curiosity won out—she opened the box and all the illnesses and hardships started coming out with hope hidden at the bottom. As Sarah became the character of Pandora, she identified the box as the Holocaust. She was terrified to open it, but realized she had to. She created a beautiful green velvet box placed on an environment of black material and ashes and filled with objects representing the Holocaust. By working through the myth of Pandora's Box she was able to open the box and take out and wear the worn yellow star her father had been forced to wear during the Holocaust, identifying him as Jewish. She also took out memorial candles which she lit honoring all the members of her family killed in the camps. After this process she felt lighter, as if a load had been lifted, and she was able to recognize the origin of her fears and nightmares and move on. She understood that her family's silence was to protect her, yet for her emotional health she needed to break the silence. Reflecting on her process, Sarah told me, "I really needed the distance provided by working outside of myself. I had many issues surrounding the Holocaust and through this process was able to get to the edge and face the fear."

Finding the Story

In the two previous exercises we began exploring creative projection and discovering our own creative DNA. We were also learning to develop and trust our intuition to guide us. To find our story we must listen carefully to our deepest inner voice and trust that the process of looking for the story is in itself important. The challenge is to let go of any assumptions as to what story we think we "want" or "like" or "believe" is right. Unfortunately, our brain loves the familiar and will keep us bound by old patterns and beliefs as the neurons are well worn and ready to fire up. However, we can counter this by remaining curious and open to discovery and surprise. If you feel stuck, one way to approach this exploration is to begin by reflecting on the images or feelings that came up in the previous two exercises (*Encounter* and *Chaos and Order*). What stays with you—a particular texture, color, movement, feeling? Whatever it is, start your search with this. For example, if your creation for chaos elicited feelings of fear or anger, look for stories that have this element. Or if your first-person story in the *Encounter* exercise had specific images and scenes, look for stories that have these. In a way your unconscious has already begun to lead you where you need to go. The messages can be subtle, hidden, and sometimes obtuse, but if you pay attention, they will be your guide.

The first step is to read or listen to a variety of different myths, fairy tales, and traditional stories, preferably from diverse cultures. Interestingly, we are often drawn to stories outside of our own culture; even though they are unfamiliar, there is some element that resonates. While we acknowledge that we cannot possibly understand the cultural or traditional context, the story itself speaks to us. As much as possible, try and find the stories in their original form. Unfortunately, Disney and others sanitized these stories to such a degree that the darker and essential elements are missing. As you browse the bookshelves or the internet, you will enter a magical world with a vast array of characters both human and not human. There may be gods, demons, monsters, mystical animals, animate objects, and sacred quests… You can also search in audio books or podcasts. You may want to experiment with reading and listening and noticing if you respond differently depending on how the story is presented. As you read through the different stories, pay attention to your inner responses to the title, illustrations, and different sections of the story. You may notice that you feel nothing for a long time and then suddenly one story brings tears, or anger, or discomfort, or spontaneous laughter. The "right" story is ultimately identified from an intuitive recognition or response that may be emotionally unsettling, or mysterious. It could be that a particular character, image, or line of text stays with you and won't go away. For some people this process of finding the story is immediate and clear, while for others, it can be confusing and frustrating. Whatever happens for you is exactly the way it should be—trust the path itself even if it has strange twists and turns. Eventually you will be led to the "right" character and story, the one that has been waiting for you to find it.

The Process for Finding Your Story

1. Explore many myths, fairy tales, and traditional stories from diverse cultures, trying to find the original versions. You can search on the internet, in bookstores, in libraries, or on audio recordings. Stay open, without any preconceptions as to what the right story is beforehand. Let yourself be surprised.

2. As you read and explore different stories, pay attention to what happens in your body. Does one story cause you to tighten your muscles, bring tears, make you angry? Notice the feelings that come up spontaneously. When you find a story that elicits a strong somatic response or an inner sense of knowing, this is your story.

3. Once you find the story in the original or the earliest version you can find, copy or write it up in your journal and read it over many times until it feels familiar. Also write about your process of finding the story. Was it an easy process, challenging, frustrating? How did you organize your search—what did you look for? What was your process of "knowing"? Did you have a somatic response, a strong feeling, an immediate intuition?

Telling the Story

Once you have found your story, it is important to tell the story to someone else. Ideally this would take place in your circle of support. If not, find someone to tell the story to. For the *Story Within* process I have designed very specific rules for the teller and the listener. When we name something, it becomes ours. Telling the story is different from reading the story. Do not use notes, but rather just say what you remember of the details of the story. It doesn't matter whether you get some details wrong or forgot a part of the story, what matters is what stays with you. When we tell a story, what we say or leave out is important. This is the beginning of the projection and our personal relationship with the story and character. It is paramount at this stage of the process that the teller of the story is not interrupted or in any way interfered with. If the listener interrupts or asks questions or tries to get clarification or corrects the details, this takes away from the teller's experience. This is a fragile and delicate moment for the teller and they can be quite vulnerable. Therefore, it is extremely important for the listener to be a silent supportive witness. The response to the telling of the story for both the teller and the listener is to give expression through the arts. Art-to-art responses establish a new way of relating where both participants are vulnerable and there is no analysis or interpretation. Essentially it becomes an art-to-art dialogue rather than a verbal or intellectual discussion. To gain the most benefit from the process, please follow the steps outlined below.

TELLING THE STORY EXERCISE

1. **Check in.** In the circle of support: before telling the story, do a check-in. Go around the circle and have each of you say a maximum of three words, or a gesture, sound, image, color, that expresses your process of finding the character and story. Make sure that each person sticks to the three-word limit!

2. **Get into pairs.** Sit comfortably across from each other so you can make easy eye contact. Choose who will go first. Explain that it is important to follow the instructions.

3. **Teller.** You as the teller have five to ten minutes to tell your story saying as much as you remember. All the specific details are not important, just say what you can about the story in the order that you remember.

4. **Listeners.** Try to be in an open and receptive state of mind. Don't worry about remembering all the details of the story, you will not have to recount them in any way. Just pay attention and allow the story and characters to enter your body and unconscious. The most important gift you can give the teller is your silent supportive presence. Do not interrupt, do not ask questions. Listen attentively and supportively. You can nod and smile when appropriate but do not express shock or sadness, etc. If you do, it can take away from the teller's experience. Accept whatever the teller says even if you know the story and they get it wrong—do not correct them! Once the teller has finished, you as the listener will ask if the teller has anything they want to add. That is it. The teller can add whatever they wish. Then the listener says, "Thank you for telling your story," and you both separate.

5. **Art-to-art responses.** The teller and the listener separate. The listener will do a response creation using whatever mediums they choose: art, drama, music, movement, or a combination; that is just their personal response to the story. This is not an analysis, or interpretation. As the listener you are just expressing how the story affected you. There is no right or wrong, just be authentic. Your personal response may elicit new information and a new perspective for the teller. Or it may be irrelevant. What is important and often moving for the teller is that something in the story touched you as the listener and that you are willing to share this internal experience creatively. Meanwhile the teller is also doing a creative expression which is their personal response to having told the story. Then both teller and listener come back together. As the listener you go first and present your creation to the teller. No interpretation or analysis, just your own personal response. Then as the teller you

share your creative piece about your experience of telling the story. Then you can both share about the process without any interpretation or analysis. As the listener you give your creation to the teller since this is about their story. If the medium was movement or drama, the teller can video you doing the creative response.

6. **Switch roles.** Now the teller becomes the listener and the listener becomes the teller and you go through the exact same process.

7. **Thank you.** When you both finish the entire process, find a way to thank each other for this sharing and then separate and write about the process in your journals.

Working with Clients

This exercise forms the beginning of the identification with the character and story. The frame of how this is introduced is essential and key to the work. The directive is *not* to choose a story or character they want to be like, but rather a story that moves them, maybe brings them to tears for a reason not understood. There is something mysterious about this story or character, but still it calls to them… This exercise reinforces the client's inner sense of "knowing" and what that means for them and how to identify it.

Art-to-art responses establish a new way of relating where both participants are vulnerable and there is no analysis or interpretations. If you are working individually with a client, you take on the role of the listener and respond through art. I would suggest that you choose a medium you are not "good" at, something a bit uncomfortable. If you are too skilled in a medium, this can be intimidating for the client. In contrast, if you respond in a medium you are less comfortable in, then you model taking risks, being imperfect, and being vulnerable, which helps your client feel they can do the same. It is important to remember in your creative response to your client telling their story that you are not interpreting or analyzing but just authentically expressing whatever aspect touched you.

Things to Watch Out For

- *Clients struggle to find a story.* Help them by looking through stories together with books or on the internet. Guide them to listen to their own responses until they have an inner sense of knowing. For some clients who have experienced trauma this can take many sessions because they are disconnected from themselves. Their disconnection may have helped them survive the trauma, and becoming reconnected may bring up fear, and strong feelings. Help them to feel safe throughout the process and tell them to take all the time they need.

- *Clients cannot decide between two stories.* For the telling exercise, have them choose one story to start with. The one they choose may lead them to their choice. Or, have them tell both stories and see what comes up in the art-to-art responses. Sometimes this choosing between two stories is an important aspect of the therapy as they may be choosing between something more accessible and familiar and something deeper and more frightening. If they can eventually take on the one that scares them, this will lead to a more in-depth discovery of their own hidden stories.

- *Clients start to intellectualize, interpret, analyze.* This is common, and often you just need to gently guide them to stay open, to try and trust the arts and the story to lead them where they need to go. And gently remind them that if they already know what the story means they will not discover anything new. This trusting of the unknown is challenging and you as the therapist need to work on that skill set so that you can be comfortable not knowing. The process of discovery is for both you and your client. Your role is to keep them safe and be a container so they can go where they need to.

My Process

Each one of us has a story waiting to be found...this is just my story... you will be led to the one for you...

Finding the Story
Check-in words: lost, curious, surprised.

> I didn't know what I was looking for but wanted something to do with chaos and order since that was a powerful exercise and elicited a lot of emotions. I started with Greek chaos and then Haida and Inuit myths and then finally searched for wild woman stories and found the story of La Loba. This stirred something in me, a visceral feeling of both attraction and discomfort...

La Loba Sings the Bones
This is based on Estés' (2008) *Women Who Run with the Wolves: Contacting the Power of the Wild Woman.*

> There is an old woman who lives in a hidden place that everyone knows in their souls but few have ever seen. She calls herself by many names. In this desert she is called La Loba. The Wolf Woman. The sole work of La Loba is the collecting of bones. She collects and preserves especially that which is in danger of being lost to the world. Her specialty is wolves. She sifts through the mountains and riverbeds looking for wolf bones, and when she has assembled an entire skeleton and the creature is laid out before her, she sits by the fire and thinks about what song she will sing. And when she is sure, she stands over the creature, raises her arms over it, and sings out. That is when the rib bones and leg bones begin to flesh out and the creature becomes furred. La Loba sings some more, and more of the creature comes into being; its tail curls upward, shaggy and strong. And La Loba sings more and the wolf creature begins to breathe.
>
> And still La Loba sings so deeply that the floor of the desert shakes, and as she sings, the wolf opens its eyes, leaps up, and runs away down the canyon. Somewhere in its running, whether by the

speed of its running, or by splashing its way into a river, or by way of a ray of sunlight or moonlight hitting it right in the side, the wolf is suddenly transformed into a laughing woman who runs free toward the horizon.

CHAPTER 11

Making a Mask

She was a beautiful young girl, kind, funny, smart, and, sadly, dying of cancer. Her parents and some of the medical staff wanted to believe she would get better and kept giving her positive messages of how well she was doing. However, when I met with her, she told me she knew she was dying and wanted to help her parents so they could talk about it. At only eight years old, she was wise beyond her years. She chose the fairy tale of "The Little Match Girl." This is a story about an impoverished young girl who is forced to go out in the freezing cold to sell matches to try and survive. As she slowly freezes to death, she lights the matches and sees beautiful visions. This young girl lying in a hospital bed, her body being destroyed by cancer, connected strongly with this story and particularly the moment when the match girl dies but also sees beautiful visions. She wanted her mask to reflect this moment, and as we made the mask, she included ashes and carefully selected images from magazines and photos of her life, and these were glued onto the mask. We arranged that her parents and older brother would come in while she was wearing the mask. Then she told them about the Little Match Girl and her beautiful visions. This was a way she could speak to her family about dying. Though her parents and brother were devastated and cried, they were also able to tell her how much they loved her and use the mask as an object to connect in a profound and authentic way. Through using the character, and particularly the mask, this young girl was able to find a way to help her traumatized family accept that she was dying and to enjoy the time she had left.

Our relationship with masks is ancient and carries a legacy of our earliest beginnings. Similar to the young girl facing death, our ancestors created masks to help them face their own mortality and their connection to the spiritual world. Even today, many cultures still use masks for healing, protection, honoring, and celebration. Part of the reason masks have stayed with us is their unique quality to be both an art form and something imbued with personal and symbolic significance. Once created, the mask becomes an integral part of performance and ritual to transmit culture and stories. Herb Rice (2019), a contemporary master carver and member of the Cowichan band, proposes, "A mask that is not danced, not used to share stories and teachings, is little more than a decorative husk." The role of creating masks is considered a sacred calling. Robert Davidson (n.d.), Haida artist, says, "When I create a new mask…I'm a medium…masks are images that shine through us from the spirit world." In ancient Greece, masks were an integral part of all theatre productions and actors wore specific masks depending on the role they played. And, as well, masks are central to Noh Theatre, a major form of classical Japanese musical drama that has been performed since the fourteenth century. I was fortunate when I was in Kyoto to see a traditional Noh performance, and despite not understanding the language or the cultural context, I felt inexplicably moved to tears by the depth of the universal and archetypal emotions being expressed. The power of masks comes through in many formats from indigenous rituals, theatre performances, Halloween, and celebrations. Currently, all over the world, masks are still used in many carnivals and ceremonies. Here is a list of just a few of them: Venetian Carnival masks, Mexican Day of the Dead masks, Chinese New Year masks, Brazilian Carnival masks, Filipino *Dinagyang* masks, African *Festima* masks, Bahamian *Junkanoo* masks, Austrian *Krampusnacht* Festival masks, Venezuelan Dancing Devils of Yare masks, Japanese *Shimokita Tengu Matsuri* masks, and there are many more.

> "Man is least himself when he speaks in his own person. Give him a mask and he will speak the truth."
>
> Oscar Wilde (1854–1900)

In art therapy and drama therapy the making of a mask is used as a therapeutic tool and can be an important way to explore the persona and the more hidden aspects of the self. In sessions clients can portray on the outside of the mask what they show to the world and express on the inside of the mask the more hidden aspects of the self (Bailey, 2007; Malchiodi, 2011). In my work with suicide survivors, those who lost loved ones to suicide, mask making allowed for a tangible expression of both the immense loss from the suicide and the effect of the shame and stigma surrounding it. Having a self-created object outside of them was important in terms of expressing their experience in a form other than words and helped to project their feelings onto something external (Silverman, 2010, 2018; Silverman, Smith, and Burns, 2013).

For the *Story Within* process, the making of the mask is a powerful way of embodying the story and character we have chosen (or that chose us) into a creative object. It is an essential first step to calling the character into our lives in a personal and meaningful way. We are entering a process both ancient and in the present moment. It can be intimidating if you have never made a mask before to know how to begin. The wonderful thing about masks is that they can be made from anything—and I mean anything. It can be something simple such as using a paper plate and painting and gluing feathers, ribbons, and other objects onto it. Or it can be more complex with a hockey or bicycle helmet as a base covered with fabric, clay, papier mâché, paint, or anything else. The possibilities are endless. It can be helpful to look up masks online or in books to get your imagination started. Below are some elements of masks that may be helpful to consider as you begin your mask making:

- Collectively, masks have been created and used cross-culturally to help communicate an understanding of the natural and supernatural.
- The mask has the capacity to both conceal and reveal at the same time. Covering the face can free behavior, allow other feelings to come through, and mean that we no longer conform to a familiar image of self.

- The mask is a potent metaphor for a meeting of the universal and the particular, immobility and change, disguise and revelation.

- The mask is an interface between the timeless world of myth and the immediate world of fact and plays a mediating role between myth and reality.

- Masks speak to us in metaphor and images. A mask can be a strong bridge between our conscious and unconscious, and the world of matter and spirit.

- Masks can be taken on and off. We become possessed by the character, then take it off, differentiating between the role and reality.

- Masks are associated with life and death, at first rigid and immobile, then coming to life when worn.

- The creative process is an intelligence that knows where it needs to go. Let the created mask evaluate itself—is it satisfied?

MAKING OF THE MASK

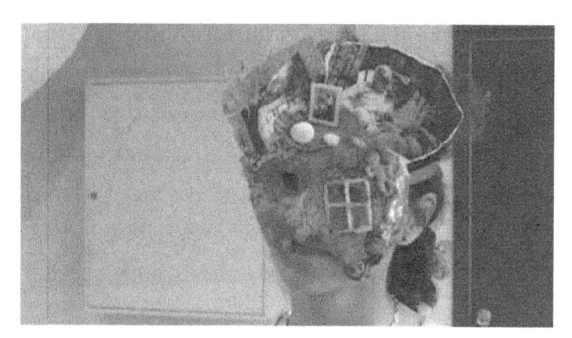

Mask by Kalie Rae

Keep in mind that the mask needs to be able to be worn in some way (directly on the face held by string tied at the back, held in front of the face with the hands, worn over the head as part of fabric…etc.). You must be able to move with it to go through the full process.

1. Clear a space in your house or find a place where you can get messy. Put plastic on surfaces and on you for protection.

2. Collect objects you want to use in your mask from around your house, recycle bins, nature, dollar stores, friends' houses, the street, etc. For example, blank masks, leaves, dirt, ashes, cotton balls, metal, wire, plastic, straw, pinecones, shells, etc. Use this as an opportunity to allow your story and character to lead you to the "right" objects and materials. It doesn't matter if you have no idea of what form the mask will take. Trust your intuition and the guidance of your character that you will find the materials you need.

3. Have all the art materials you need such as paint, brushes, glue (glue gun if you are comfortable with this), stapler, hole puncher, papier mâché, clay, etc.

4. Put on music (if helpful) and let the choice of music be determined by your character and by your intuition. Take a moment to be quiet and ask for guidance from something deep within or beyond you so that the mask comes through you. This is your personal ritual to get started, so find a way to let go of all your other demands and busy life to focus on this process.

5. Begin assembling the materials you want in the form that feels right. It is okay to try many different shapes and materials—that is part of the process. Some of you will have an image of what the mask should look like and others will only find out when you are working with the material. Trust your own creative DNA and know that the process of making the mask is just as important as the final form, so whatever you experience, know that it is teaching you something about your character.

6. Continue to work on your mask until it feels finished. This may take hours or days. You may need to let your mask dry and then add more materials, or you may need to take a break and then come back to your mask to see it fresh. Take all the time you need so that you feel satisfied that the mask in some way

expresses your story and character. Please remember not to judge or to have any expectations about how it "should" look. There is no right or wrong way to do this and the goal is *not* to make a "pretty" mask but rather to make one that speaks to you and will help you in some way to connect with your character. It might be best to keep your mask to yourself, or only share it with friends and family who will not make judgments or express their own interpretation. Hearing feedback from others at this point can be destructive and distract from your own process.

7. Decide where and how you want to store the mask. This is important. Does it need a box, to be covered, or to be displayed and seen?

8. When you are finished, take some time to look at your mask and do a creative response to seeing the finished mask. This creative response can be in any medium and can be something quick and spontaneous. Then write in your journal about the process of making your mask. What was the process from beginning to end? How did you find the materials and what did you end up using? What was challenging about the process? What was satisfying? How did you feel before, during, and after the process? How do you feel now about the mask?

Working with Clients

When working with clients, they can make the mask at home if they are capable. If they carry through with the exercises and the projection out of the sessions, it deepens both the projection and the therapeutic alliance. It gives them a reason to link with the therapy outside of sessions and creates a transition from real life to the therapy session. If working in a group, when clients share their masks, they get to know each other's characters and the masks become part of the group and the sessions. Using the mask as both an object (placed in the room) and subject (worn and embodied) sets this up as a frame to work with throughout the sessions (see Chapter 12, "Placing and Embodying the Mask," for more details). Therapeutically, the process of creating the mask is just as important as the final product. It is helpful to ask clients how they made their creative decisions on the use of materials and what worked and what did not, and the feeling state throughout the process.

Things to Watch Out For

- *Clients are not able to make the mask by themselves.* You can have them work on the mask in the sessions. Have materials available (these do not have to be elaborate) and introduce them to the various materials and ask them what they are personally drawn to and what their character is drawn to. You are helping them connect with their intuition and with the character. This can take several sessions, and your encouragement and presence provide the safety they need to continue.

- *A client becomes overwhelmed when making the mask.* If they are making the mask at home, caution them if it feels overwhelming to stop and bring the mask to the session. If working on the mask in the sessions, also stop the process. Since the mask can be an object, this is when you can ask them directly what would make the mask feel safer. They may want to cover the mask or just cover the eyes or keep the mask far away from them. Allow them to determine what they need and help them to enact this. Once the mask feels safer, ask if they want to continue working on creating the mask. It may be that they cannot and will continue to work with the mask as an object separate from themselves until they are ready to gradually bring the mask closer (please see discussion of the mask as an object in Chapter 12, "Placing and Embodying the Mask").

My Process

I put on music and moved around the room with my eyes closed. Immediately I became La Loba. She was holding her head, exhausted, roaming the earth looking for bones, alone, burdened, in the wilds. It felt very ancient and powerful...

What do I see when I look at my mask? Something connected to nature yet magical, other worldly, not fully human. Twigs coming through her life, coming through her... She looks old, exhausted, mouth is formed for singing. She scares me, but I am drawn to her...

CHAPTER 12

Placing and Embodying the Mask

She walked into the room like a shadow, completely silent and not taking up any space. Making no eye contact, she quickly sat down slumped in a chair. The medical staff knew her as the beautiful ten-year-old with the long red hair who never spoke; this was clinically referred to as "selectively mute." She had not spoken a word for six months and no one knew why. Her family was baffled, and according to the medical experts nothing was physically wrong. In our work together she chose the story of "The Little Mermaid" who gives her voice to the witch in exchange for the love of the prince. When she found this story, it was validating to find a character who, like herself, had chosen to give up her voice. She made a mask using a pair of black tights filled with newspaper with glued-on images of female models and superstars. The images were cut up and ripped apart. The mouth was covered with masking tape. When she placed the mask in the room, she put it under a chair with plastic wrap around it so you could see it, but it was covered and protected. She became very emotional when she stood back and looked at her mask. We communicated through writing and she wrote that the mermaid looked incredibly sad and alone. When she put on the mask and embodied the Little Mermaid she glided through the room and settled in a corner, making herself as small as possible. Then she started crying, making gasping sounds. I picked a few percussion instruments and sat with her in her corner and asked if she could play the mermaid's sadness with an instrument. She grabbed a small drum and started banging on it, getting louder and louder, until at one point she also began very quietly using her voice to make guttural sounds. Eventually her voice became stronger. Over the next few sessions we worked with percussion and sounds until she gradually started to whisper to me and told me the story of how she was being bullied in school and over the internet. Once she allowed me to disclose this to her parents, they were able to tell the school and decided to move her to a new school. In her new school she started speaking again, at first very softly, but she slowly regained her confidence. In our last session she told me, "Seeing the mask of the Little Mermaid so sad and alone released my own feelings, and then becoming the character myself, I realized how I had given up and basically didn't want to exist anymore. Even though I chose this character because I identified with her not speaking, she gave me my voice back."

Once a mask is created it begins to take on a life of its own. As an object it is already imbued with personal meaning and feelings. However, to truly explore the character, it is necessary to begin working with the mask as both an object and a subject. As an object it can be placed in the room, lifted up, spoken to, and witnessed. As a subject it is worn and embodied. Having both options allows us to negotiate between a strong emotional identification (when worn) and more emotional distance (when placed in the room outside of the self). Masks can capture any state of mind. They evoke, reveal, and conceal all at the same time. Even the most simply constructed masks can powerfully transform the face and come to life when worn. The mask becomes charged with a vital force from within both the wearer and the character. Creating and wearing a mask is often used in art therapy as a way of exploring or uncovering difficult emotions. Melissa Walker, an art therapist who worked with veterans suffering from PTSD, found that creating and wearing the masks helped give the veterans a voice to express their trauma (Stone, 2015). Even without the wounds of war, most of us have learned to disguise and repress aspects of ourselves that are not approved of, such as anger, greed, envy, and jealousy. We also may repress positive traits such as creativity, exuberance, or confidence when these qualities are not appreciated in our environment. As we explore our mask and character, we may also reclaim our inherent creativity, working with art, drama, sound, and movement.

In the *Story Within* process, after choosing the story and character and making the mask, it is necessary to embark on the task of invoking and embodying the role. This is an essential process both in traditional theatre and in drama therapy. Stanislavsky (1961) and Meisner and Longwell (1987) describe the value, in performance, of using perceptual senses, memories, and past experiences when embodying a character to create emotional truth on stage. The process of entering into the role of the character is an essential therapeutic process in drama therapy. As Landy (1993) proposes, "The invocation of the role…is a calling into being of that part of the person that will inspire a creative search for meaning" (p.47). Paradoxically, as we work with a fictional character, we are actually coming closer to our own hidden inner world. As Jennings (1990), a pioneer drama therapist, points out, "the nearer we work to a person's own life, i.e. the more proximity, the more limitations we impose on the exploration of their life story. The greater the dramatic distance we create, the greater the range of therapeutic choices available" (p.111). It is often during the exercise *Placing and Embodying the Mask* that the relationship with the character deepens and the character comes alive and develops a voice of its own.

INTRODUCTION OF MASKS

Mask Warm-Up
If working with your circle of support, each person introduces their mask to the group in whatever way feels right for them. You can put it on, hold it, stand in the center, or put the mask in the center of the circle. Keep it brief. While you introduce your mask, say the name of your story and character. The group all repeat the story and character's name.

Placing the Mask in the Room
1. *Placement.* Find a place in the room to place your mask. Let your mask lead you to where it wants to be in the room, whether on

a windowsill, under a chair or table, or hanging from the ceiling. Place the mask in the right position as to where it wants to face. You can use fabrics, pillows, chairs, mats, stones, feathers, etc. to be part of how your mask wants to be placed. For example, you may want to place the mask on a stool with fabric draped over the stool and other objects next to the mask and stones leading up to it. Check the height, placement, arrangement, and colors, and get some distance and look at it from many angles.

2. *Response.* Once the placement and what surrounds it feels right and complete, step away and do a quick response to it through any medium you choose (movement, sound, drama, art, poetry).

3. *Journal.* Then write in your journal about the experience of placing it in the room and what you see when you look at it now. Please try to refrain from analysis or interpretation; stay with what you see and how it makes you feel.

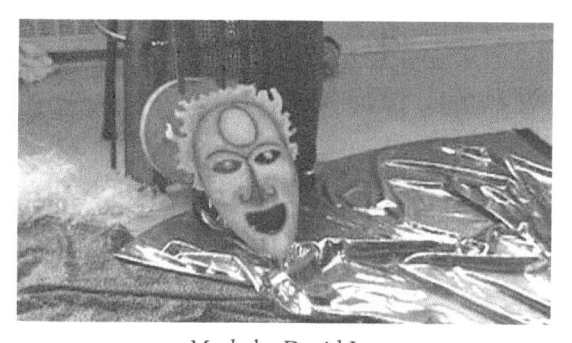

Masks by David Jan

Embodiment

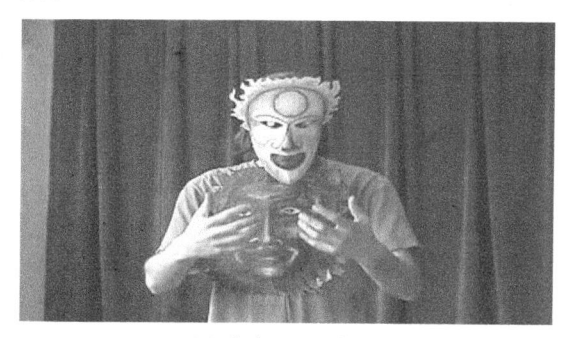

Masks by David Jan

1. Stand up, put your journal away, and find a way to approach your mask physically. Let your body be the guide as to how you approach the mask. Do you face the mask directly or face away? Do you move slowly or quickly? Are you at the same level as the mask or below or above it? Spend time with this until you are close to your mask.

2. Slowly pick up the mask and spend a moment looking into the eyes of your mask. See if you can feel your mask looking back at you. When you are ready, put the mask on. Let yourself feel the mask on your body and let the mask begin to transform your body, mind, spirit, into the character. Feel your breathing change, your body change, your arms, legs, etc., transform, take on the shape, weight, consistency of your character. Pay attention to your sense of weight: does your character move with a heavy or light quality? Does it sink into the ground, or float free? What is the tension in your character's body? Is it bound and very tense and hard to move, or is it free-flowing and loose? Does your character approach things directly with a strong focus, or indirectly with no specific focus? Does your character take up a lot of space and take large steps, or take up little space with tiny steps? What level does it move on, crawling, walking, slithering? Where does your character like to go in the room? See how much you can let yourself become your character through movement.

3. As you move as your character, let the sounds your character makes come through you. Does your character sing, growl, speak, whistle, moan, or is your character silent?

4. Let your character begin to interact with the objects in the room—walls, curtains, rug, floor, chairs, blackboard, materials. Choose one object you find in the room that your character wants to interact with and begin to interact with it. The interaction could be angry, loving, careless. What does this object mean to your character? Then move with this object around the room.

Placing and Embodying the Mask   143

5. With your circle of support, begin to interact with the other characters in the room. As your character, interact through movement, sound, or words. Try not to break out of your character and role and do not interact as yourself.

6. After interacting for a while, let your character begin to concentrate on the task it needs to accomplish. For example, it could be to run away from a monster or enemy, find a treasure, or save a loved one. Be aware of other characters around you and, if it feels right for your character, try to get the other characters to help you with your task. But remember that all of you must stay in the role of your character. If your character is solitary and would not ask others for help or help others—do not engage for the sake of this prompt.

7. As you try and do your task, find another object (or the same one) to help with your character's journey and task. Also find a word, sound, or song to help.

8. To end this embodiment process, find a place in the room that feels right and find a still posture that expresses your character in this moment. After holding the posture, take a few deep breaths: slowly relax, come out of the role, and take the mask off.

9. Bring the mask back to its original home and see if that placement and the surrounding objects still feel right. If not, make the necessary changes. Does your mask now want to change positions, levels, where it's facing, etc.?

10. De-role: get out of your character. Shake it off and spend a moment stretching and feeling in your own body.

11. Write in your journal about the entire process. What was it like to place the mask in the room? What was challenging and what was rewarding? How did you feel when you saw the mask in its home? How did your body change when you embodied your character? What did it feel like to move through the room as your character? What feelings and sensations came up? What

were your chosen objects and how did your character interact with them? How did you as your character interact with other characters? Were you aggressive, passive, fearful, flirtatious, loving? What did you learn about your character? What was more challenging or satisfying, the placement of the mask or the embodying part? Did anything come up that was surprising?

Working with Clients

For some clients the placing of the mask will be satisfying and meaningful, but they will have trouble with physically embodying their character. For others, the placement will be quick and meaningless, but the embodiment is what really moves them. This is an effective way for your client to discover more about their creative DNA and what creative mediums and perceptions are more natural. For those who are very visual, the placement may land deeply, while for those more kinesthetic, the movement will make the character more alive. When the members of a group interact as their characters they get to know more about their own character through the interaction and it creates alliances and bonds within the group at an unconscious and archetypal level. If you work individually then you are the witness as your client places the mask and moves as their character.

Things to Watch Out For

- *A client is not able to place their mask in the room.* Help them do this by walking around with them and ask them questions about where the mask might want to be. Have them try various places and positions and stay beside them.

- *A client is not able to embody the character: they are over-distanced.* If they have trouble getting into the role of their character, help them put on the mask and ask them to find one posture or one movement that would express their character. If this is too challenging, have them teach it to you and they can look at it on you and then try it themselves.

Once they have one posture or movement then you can help them expand this into more movements and sounds.

- *A client is not able to embody the character: they are under-distanced.* If it is too overwhelming to put on the mask and embody their character, have them direct you holding the mask and moving with it. They can continue to direct your movements and sounds and stay as the director, maintaining a safer and more distant stance. Or, if they become more comfortable, they could hold the mask away from their face and move as their character.

Homework

Find or make a costume for your character. This may happen at the same time as making your mask and may be an integral part of the mask. Or, you may only start to work on it after the mask is made and you have embodied it. You can use fabric that you already have or sew together varied materials. You can also use objects as part of your costume such as shields, swords, shells, pieces of glass, photos—the sky is the limit! Have fun and use your imagination. Let your character guide you.

My Process
Placement of My Mask

> I was immediately drawn to my Doumbek drum and placed the mask on top of the drum with gold sparkling material flowing down to the floor where I placed stones of varying sizes and shapes.

> What do I see? La Loba looks as if she is singing—the rocks keep her connected to the earth. The sparkles in the material reflect the sparkles in the mask. I feel fear, reverence, and trust that she knows what she is doing...

Embodiment

I feel shaky as if I entered another reality. La Loba is powerful and can bring the dead to life. Her task is to gather the bones—no one can help her. She still scares me, but I love that I opened her mouth so she can sing…

CHAPTER 13

Finding the Moment

Sam was court-ordered into a high-risk youth program as an alternative to prison. At the age of 18 he had an extensive criminal record, an accusation of inappropriate sexual behavior with his sister, and a history of gang-related violence. He was six feet tall, muscular, and defiant. He was also an excellent rap singer. We worked with rap. He chose the story of Jack and the Beanstalk. He said he always liked this story because Jack "makes out okay in the end with the money." Through our work together Sam was able to embody the character of Jack and rap about his story and his fears about the giant. One day I suggested working with climbing the beanstalk. We used a ladder, and as he was climbing, he suddenly stopped and started shaking. Eventually he disclosed that when he was a child his father had sexually abused him in the attic. He had forgotten the abuse (his father left when he was seven), but in the act of climbing the beanstalk to face the giant he re-experienced climbing the steps to face his father in the attic. From this point on Sam began to work with facing his own abuse, his abuse of his sister, and his own fears about gang violence. He reconciled with his family and was able to leave the gang. During his last session he reflected on his process and said, "Fairy tales, yeah, right, like I really believed this sh-t, but hey, climbing that beanstalk led me to my old man, the giant mother f-cker, hard stuff, but I'm glad I did this, it changed my life…" The last time I heard from him he was sending out demos of his rap music.

Each myth, fairy tale, or traditional story has many specific and unique moments. For example, even in a story as short and simple as "The Three Little Pigs," there are distinct dramatic situations, each one conveying different emotions, relationships, and themes. Let's take the scene of one little pig placing the first brick to build their house and juxtapose it with the wolf falling down the chimney into the pot of oil. These moments take place in one short story and yet they are miles apart in terms of character, feelings, and actions. In the *Story Within* process, once clients have chosen their character and story, they are asked to focus on a specific moment within the story they feel most drawn to. It is not necessarily the moment they want or aspire to, but the moment that stays with them, so that when they read that scene they are strongly affected. For one of my clients, the moment before Alice steps through the looking glass provided a metaphor for her fear of the unknown. For another young woman, it was the process of identifying the moment when Snow White discovers she had been poisoned by her stepmother (the Queen disguised as an old woman) that allowed her to work through a difficult separation process from her own depressed mother. Therefore, the process of choosing a specific moment in the story can become a catalyst for discovering the essence of the character's inner conflicts and emotional struggles. This can often lead to insights and personal connections and discoveries. If there is not a commitment to one specific moment in the story, the process will not progress into the final stages.

FINDING THE MOMENT EXERCISE

Preparation

For some of you the moment may come immediately, perhaps even when you first choose the story. However, for others it might be a challenge and take time to discover.

The mask embodiment exercise is often a catalyst for finding the moment. What was your character doing? What were the movements? Did they encounter something or someone? What aspects of the story were most present? Were they engaged in a specific task? If the moment did not come with the mask embodiment exercise, then it should become clear in the next exercise, *Soundscape*.

If you are still struggling to find your moment, try the following. Read through the story again. Go through your journal and look at the themes and moments that have come up already in the mask making and embodying.

Finding the Moment

1. Choose one moment in your story that you are strongly affected by. It is important that you don't try and analyze the rationale for choosing this moment. It is actually much more powerful and ultimately profound to maintain a sense of not knowing and allow the moment to choose you. Trust that it will lead you to where you need to go.

2. The moment can be extremely short, for example when the wolf in "The Three Little Pigs" is looking down at the pot of boiling oil he is heading towards, or when Humpty Dumpty falls off the wall and shatters. Or it can be longer, for example the moment in the story of the Selkie when the hunter finds the seal coat of the seal woman, steals it, and then goes to hide it, or the moment when Persephone is abducted by Hades and is taken down into the underworld. It can be any moment in the story that stays with you and affects you in some way when you read it.

3. The moment should not contain more than one to three dramatic actions. Two examples include: (1) The wolf sees the pot of oil, the wolf is falling towards the oil; (2) Persephone is taken by Hades, rides in the chariot to Hades, and enters Hades.

4. It is very helpful to have the specific moment chosen before the *Soundscape* exercise and it is essential before the exercise following that, the *Environment*.

Working with Clients

Finding the moment can be a difficult task for the client. It entails an ability to focus and make choices. Also, it brings the client closer to the essence of their personal connection to the story. This can bring excitement or fear and resistance. It is important to reassure them that they will be exploring this moment in a safe and creative way.

Things to Watch Out For

- *A client cannot choose a moment.* If they are struggling to choose, go through the different moments in the story with them and watch for their somatic reactions. Ask them about their reactions and how they respond to the different moments. Usually with the therapist's help, clients will eventually be able to choose a moment.

- *A client is overwhelmed by a chosen moment.* Help them find one part of the moment that feels safe. Or some object, quality, or character in the moment that is helpful and safe and focus on this aspect until they are ready to explore the whole moment. You can also have them explore the moment with more distance using the mask as an object or directing someone else as the character in a later exercise.

- *A client is not connecting with the chosen moment.* You can help explore other moment possibilities as perhaps the moment they chose is not really the right moment for them. Sometimes clients go through several moments before they find the right one. Or if they want to stay with this moment, help them embody the moment wearing the mask and help them engage with the task and movement of the character in this specific moment.

My Moment

La Loba singing over the bones when they start to come to life…

CHAPTER 14

Soundscape

He was pacing the halls of the psychiatric ward. A large man, bald, who was muttering loudly to himself and shaking his fist at other patients. I approached him slowly and started to walk beside him. He tolerated my presence and then turned to me and asked, "Why are you following me?" I smiled and said, "I'm here to create something together." He asked, "Why?" and I said, "Why not?" He nodded and he said, "Okay." We went into the creative arts therapy room and we were the only ones there. He was not interested in any art materials, didn't want to sit down, and continued to pace in this room. I had brought some instruments with me and brought out a round animal skin drum and started playing it with a mallet, a steady heartbeat-type rhythm while I walked beside him. He slowed down his steps and started making a low guttural sound in the rhythm of the drum. Then he reached for the drum and I gave it to him, and he played the same rhythm but a bit louder. I started singing softly what felt like an ancient melody and he joined me. Our walking became a circle around the circumference of the room, and as we continued to do this he became calmer and calmer until we stood together in silence. Then he sat down and began working with clay. As he molded the clay, he told me about his visions and voices and how hard it was to get them to stop. They would stop when he was on medication but then he felt everything was dull and muted. He created a bowl from the clay and put colored marbles inside and said that was his brain—too many marbles... We both laughed and he looked over at the drum and smiled, saying, "I liked that sound stuff—made me feel better as if I knew what to do and where to go..."

As we go through life we are bombarded by sounds: traffic, dogs barking, lawn mowers, the wind in the trees, people laughing. Much of the time we don't pay attention and consider this as background noise. However, this is our daily "soundscape," the hearable elements of our environment. We can consider a soundscape as analogous to a landscape. A landscape includes a broad view of everything you can see around you such as trees, grass, rivers, buildings, streets. Similarly, a soundscape includes the audible experience of a place, an event, or a specific environment. We appreciate the aesthetic variety in our landscape, whether it is the light reflecting off the ocean, the red of the New Mexico hills, or the sight of a tall building against the sky. If we stop and listen, we can also appreciate the aesthetic quality of our audible environment or soundscape.

Many music therapists use the idea of a soundscape in their clinical and community work. One common exercise is when one member of the group acts as conductor, whilst the rest of the group are the "orchestra." Using their voices (and body percussion or instruments, if appropriate), the group expresses a soundscape of a theme or mood presented by the conductor. This communication through music allows for a more direct emotional exchange than through verbal communication (Bieleninik *et al.*, 2017). The link between sound and healing goes back to ancient times and currently there are several music therapists who are researching the idea of the soundscape in hospitals and how the environmental sounds to which patients are exposed can affect their healing (Weymann, 2018). It would certainly be different to go into a hospital and have healing sounds rather than the cacophony of machines beeping! Cultural anthropology is another field that has studied the concept of sound(scape) since the late 1960s using a range of equipment to record the sounds inherent in different communities and cultures. It is clear that we are affected by sounds and that the notion of capturing our environmental sounds and creating expressive sounds is an important aspect of healing and research.

For the *Story Within* process, the *Soundscape* exercise offers an opportunity to capture the environment of your character through sound. If you are working in a group, this exercise really establishes the idea of group support and how each person in the circle contributes something unique. It also gives each participant a chance to be the conductor, to create music, and to direct others. It is empowering for the conductor and for the musicians since each person is necessary for the soundscape to work. In individual work the client will direct the therapist, or they can record their own sounds and play them back. This exercise introduces the auditory as a primary way of knowing or feeling the character. For some people this will be an essential way in, and for others it will be more challenging.

SOUNDSCAPE EXERCISE

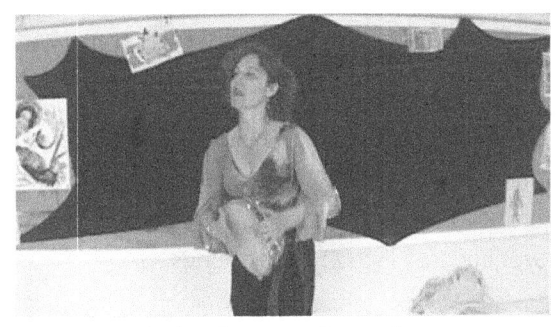

Yehudit Silverman playing drum

Preparation
Space
You need to have space so that you can sit in a circle with instruments.

Materials
Have instruments available (percussion, pots and pans, mallets, shakers, bells, recorders, and anything else you have available). As well as these, have tissue paper, scissors, rocks, and other objects. Anything that can make an interesting sound—the more options available, the better! Have your mask available so you can wear it when listening to your soundscape.

Important Note
You do not have to have any musical training to be the conductor or one of the musicians as part of the soundscape. This is not a performance and

is not about showing your skill but rather it is about serving the needs of the director so that the sounds of their character come to life.

When being part of someone else's soundscape you can refuse to do what is asked of you (play a certain instrument or make a certain sound) if you really think you cannot produce what is requested. However, the goal is to try your best and take risks in the service of something larger.

Warm-Up

1. If you are in a circle of support, have each person choose one instrument from what is available and go around the circle and have each person express how they are feeling through that instrument. This sets up the listening and attention to the auditory.

2. Then someone starts a rhythm, and everyone joins in with their instruments trying to be in the same rhythm. Walk in a circle around the room with eyes open, then stop moving and close your eyes and just listen to the sounds.

3. Keep playing your instruments and come back to your circle and get quieter and quieter until there is no sound but you still hear the rhythm inside your head. Then put the instruments either in the center of the circle or someplace accessible in the room.

The Exercise

1. Spend a few moments thinking about your character and what kinds of sounds they would hear. Then get up and let everyone explore the available instruments, so you know what they sound like.

2. Sit back down in the circle and one at a time each person gets up to be the conductor of a soundscape for their character. You as the conductor choose the instruments you want and remember that you can use objects to make sounds: rocks, scissors, staplers, tissue paper, etc. Once you decide on your instruments, hand them out to whoever you want to play them.

You can also have your circle make sounds, sing, or say words; you are free to experiment and create whatever feels right. It doesn't matter if you have no musical training; there is no right or wrong. The goal is for you to have an opportunity to create the sounds that best express your character—what they hear—what expresses the story, the feelings, etc. Experiment with listening to the instruments as they are played and direct your circle to produce the kind of sound you want.

3. Give the group a very brief description (a few sentences) of your story and the moment so they can try to capture it. Then decide on the tempo (how fast or slow), volume (loud or soft), and quality (gentle, soothing, angry, startling). Once this is set, direct your circle in the order you want the instruments (and other sounds) played and determine how the soundscape will begin and end.

4. Once the sounds feel right to you, go into the center of the circle, put on your mask, close your eyes, and just listen. It is important that you have an opportunity to be the listener and let the others be your character's soundscape.

5. Once you have had a turn as the director, take a moment to write in your journal about what came up for you, then return to the circle to take part in someone else's soundscape.

Working with Clients

If working with a group, this exercise is important to establish a sense of inclusion and group cohesion. Since each person is necessary to make the soundscape work, it offers an opportunity for all the members to feel a sense of belonging and a group identity. It also gives each participant a chance to be the conductor, to make clear creative decisions, and direct others. This can be both challenging and transformative, especially for those who have never felt empowered. In individual work the client can direct you and can also use a recorder to record other sounds, so that the soundscape is fuller. This exercise introduces the auditory as a primary way of knowing or feeling the character, and for you this may not be your primary perception, but for your client this may be natural and familiar (see Chapter 3, "Creative DNA and Perception Differences").

Things to Watch Out For

- *A client is intimidated by the instruments and is not able to create a soundscape.* Help them by introducing them to each instrument and both of you can try out the different sounds together. While doing this you can encourage your client to express what they are drawn to and what sounds feel connected to their character.

- *A client is not able to be a part of someone else's soundscape; they are refusing to participate.* You need to reiterate instructions that clients have the right to say no to a conductor if they feel they cannot produce the sounds the director is looking for. However, encourage them to try and find a way to participate. This exercise is as much for the musicians in the soundscape as for the director.

- *A client is interfering with the director and is not able to take directions.* You need to stop them and remind the group that when each person is the director all decisions are made by the director and the role of the musician is to serve as the soundscape of the character.

Homework

- Finding the moment: if you have not found your moment, please do so.
- Gather objects and materials for creating the *Environment* (next exercise).

My Process

I directed my circle of support—one woman played a goatskin round drum as a steady heartbeat, someone else shook ankle bells, and someone else played the wooden flute, alternated with primal singing. Lastly, I had two people moving rocks in their hands and dropping them on the floor.

It was powerful—I could feel myself as La Loba—when I heard the flute, I saw the expanse of land all around me, the wide plains and hills of New Mexico, and the endless sky… I was alone but not lonely… I felt nourished by the land… When I heard the rocks (bones), my body started shaking; it was very visceral and moving…

From the beginning I felt close to tears. The singing was a bit too soft, but I could hear it faintly. Perhaps this is where I am…the singing is too soft so the wolf cannot be brought to life…

CHAPTER 15

Environment

When I read his hospital chart, I was concerned about being alone with him. He was diagnosed with paranoid schizophrenia and had a history of violence. I was pregnant at the time and felt vulnerable. However, he was referred by the psychiatric team to do individual work with me and I decided at least to meet with him. As it turned out we got along really well, and he was very solicitous and gentle with me. He had little affect and tended to stare without blinking while we were in conversation. This was a bit intense, but he was committed to working on his issues around anger through the medium of the arts. He chose the story and character of the Snow Queen and he built the environment out of styrofoam and plastic wrap which he called ice. He stood inside the structure and there were no doors or windows and no way of getting out. When I asked him what it felt like to be in this environment, he said he felt "isolated, alone, and disconnected from the world." Then I inquired how he would get out and he punched a hole in the structure. Right after he did that, he stopped, looked at the damage to the environment, and told me, "I guess that's the only way I know how to get free—to make connection—to break through..." It was the building of the environment and his physical attempt to break free of it that allowed him to gain perspective and insight into his violent behavior. After this session he was able to make progress, he went back on some medication and vitamins, was able to control his symptoms, and went back to his job.

When we think of the word "environment," what comes to mind? Does it evoke images of climate change, of different plants and animals, or our own home? Originally from the French word *"environ"* meaning "surrounding," it has come to mean both the macro and micro idea of home, whether it is the cosmos, Earth, or our own living room. All living creatures have a place of residence or refuge and comfort. It is usually a setting in which an animal or human can rest and be able to store belongings. However, environment can also mean the conditions or circumstances that surround a situation or home. In terms of the *Story Within* process, each character that we work with lives in a unique environment surrounded by specific textures, landscapes, colors, sounds, and objects. Also our character has a particular relationship with their world whether they live in fear, in courage, in oblivion, or in anger. For example, Cinderella is a popular story that features a girl who is mistreated by her stepmother and stepsisters. To try and change her situation she makes a wish to a fairy godmother (in one version) or a hazel tree at her dead mother's grave (in another version). Interestingly, she does not wish to be rid of the terrible situation she is in but instead wishes to have clothes to go to the ball. What is her relationship to the world, her expectations, her sense of self? She goes to the ball but then returns to the same terrible situation with her family. Her sense of the world at first does not include the option of getting out of her bad situation. It is only when she experiences something different at the ball, is found by the prince and the glass slipper fits, that she is able to leave and start a new life. Often what we find difficult about these stories is that the character is stuck, or miserable, or struggling without seeing a way out. However, this is also what makes these stories profound and parallel with our own lives as we are often stuck in bad situations both internal and external. Working with the exercise of the environment allows us to experience in a direct way the world our character lives in. As we make a structure that in some way expresses our character's world, particularly in the moment we chose, and then embody this world, we have entered into another reality.

There are two different ways of working with your character's environment. One is to create a life-size structure that you actually enter as your character and experience what it feels like to be inside. This is the environment as "subject." In contrast, you can create a small-size environment that stays outside of your body and this is environment as "object." Having the possibility of working with the character's environment as both subject and object allows for a negotiation of distance. If the large environment is overwhelming, you can work with the small environment outside of the body. This is particularly useful when working with trauma and provides a safe and tangible way of addressing a challenging or even horrific environment. It is your character's environment, therefore there is always the safety that working with fiction and story can provide.

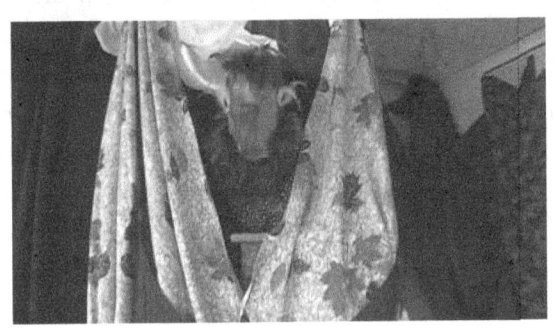

Environment by Kalie Rae

LIFE-SIZE ENVIRONMENT EXERCISE

Preparation
You need enough space to create a large structure. If you are doing this in a group, you need a large enough space for several structures to be built. The structure needs to be big enough for you to go inside.

Materials
Fabrics of many textures, colors, sizes, objects that relate to your character, chairs or table to use as the base for your structure, yarn, paint, tea lights, mirrors, whatever you have collected.

Instruments
Percussion or any other instrument that is appropriate for your character.

The Exercise
1. Group check-in. Share one object you brought in for your environment. Briefly share whatever you want to about the object.

2. Then begin to walk around the room feeling your posture, movements, breathing, sounds, and sense of weight as you become your character. Let your character guide you as to where in the room to set up your structure.

3. Once you have found your place then begin to build the structure. It can be fabric that is draped over chairs or hung from the ceiling or from the wall. It can be completely closed or open on the top and sides. There is no right or wrong way to build it. The important aspect is that it truly expresses your character in the moment that you chose (or that chose you).

4. Use materials that you brought from home, or what is available in the space. You can use feathers, stones, cotton, straw, blankets, pillows, rugs, lights, chimes, branches, dirt, moss, ashes, whatever feels authentic for your character. It doesn't matter if the environment or the materials makes sense or that you "understand" it. What is important is that in some way the structure you build gives you a visceral and direct experience of your character.

5. Decide how you will get in and out of your structure. You need to be able to go into your structure and stay inside it.

6. Once the structure feels right, go inside and see if it needs anything else. If so, find and add what is needed. Then go and get your mask and costume and put them on and enter your character's environment. How does your character like to enter their environment? Is there a ritual that is necessary before entering?

7. Once you are inside the environment with your mask and costume on, embody your character in their environment. What does your character do in their environment? Are they singing, sighing, mumbling, working, hiding, plotting? What are the sounds, the colors, the movements of your character? How does your character explore their world?

8. If you are working in a group, then decide on a time factor and when you will all end the environment exploration. When the time is up, leave your environments, take off your masks, and go as a group to each environment and meet each character. When you get to your character's environment, put on your mask and costume and introduce your character in the first person and say a line or two or a sound. Decide how you want the group to witness you in your environment. How close do you want them? When you are finished, take off your mask and costume and de-role to shake the character off.

9. The group will respond to each person's environment with a movement sculpt (a gestural pose or stance that is either still or moving and can include a sound or word). This sculpt is an authentic personal response to witnessing the group member in their character's environment. The role of the witnesses is to be supportive and hold the space but not to comment on the environment. The group can do the response all together or one at a time. Then move on to the next character and environment.

If you are doing this in your personal therapy with another professional, have your therapist be the witness and they can do the response. If you are doing this alone, find a trusted friend to be your witness.

SMALL-SIZE ENVIRONMENT EXERCISE

Preparation

You just need enough space to create a small object outside your body. If you are doing this with a group, you need enough space so all of you can create small objects.

Materials

You will need different size containers: boxes (jewelry size, tea container size, candy size, tissue box size, pill box size), bowls (plastic, wooden), yogurt containers (big and small), jars (of different sizes and shapes), ribbons, yarn, tissue paper, felt, paint, markers, glitter, marbles, rocks, feathers, cotton, glue, tape, stapler, etc.

The Exercise

1. Let your character guide you to choose a container from what is available that feels right to express your character's environment and moment.

2. Once you have your container, then use materials such as paint, feathers, clay, glitter, dirt, etc. to express your moment inside and outside of the small container.

3. Once the small container is made, look at it and give it a title and a sentence, and respond to it through movement and sound.

4. Find a partner or discuss with everyone in your group.

5. Then write about the entire process (life-size environment and small-size environment) in your journal.

Life-Size Environment: Questions for Reflection

- What was the process of building the life-size environment like? Was it easy, quick, a challenge; did things break or fall down?

- What was it like to be inside the life-size environment? Was it comfortable, claustrophobic, freeing? What was the feeling state? Did you as your character want to stay in the environment or get out? What did your character do in their environment?

- Did the large environment bring you closer to your character? If so, in what way?

- Was anything surprising?

- Did you have any insights about your character? If so, when and how?

Small-Size Environment: Questions for Reflection

- What was the process like of building the small-size environment? Was it easy, quick, a challenge; did things break or fall down?
- What was it like to witness the inside and outside of the small-size environment? Was it satisfying, uncomfortable, emotional? What was the feeling state?
- Did the small environment bring you closer to your character?
- Was anything surprising?
- Did you have any insights about your character? If so, when and how?

Working with Clients

It can be an important therapeutic process for the client to struggle in creating the environment for their character. Sometimes as therapists we want to "fix" and "help" so that our client is less stressed. As they wrestle with trying to get their structure to work, we may become uncomfortable, and as a way of dealing with our own discomfort we intervene. However, if we can learn to embrace the discomfort and challenges of our clients, we can truly help them discover their own agency and solutions. As therapists we are the container for the client's experience, and we need to support whatever is emerging and trust that even if the environment falls apart time after time this is what they need to go through. Perhaps this falling apart is an inherent part of their character and also of their own lives.

Things to Watch Out For

- *A client is not able to make their life-size environment.*
  Walk with them around the room and ask them to try out various places in the room to see if it feels right. Then help them choose material. Don't make suggestions, but rather

encourage them to pick up and explore different materials and ask them which one feels best. Stay beside them for the entire process and they can direct you to help them build the structure. Work beside them under their direction.

- *A client becomes overwhelmed in their character's environment.* Help the client to come out of the environment and de-role, paying particular attention to them feeling their feet on the ground, breathing, and being back in their own body. You can work with them using the life-size environment as object—sitting away from it but looking at it, responding to it through different mediums. Or, if this is too much, you can go directly to the small-size environment which may be less overwhelming.

- *A client is not able to connect with their character in their environment.* Help them to find the right movements, sounds, tasks for their environment. Help them focus on one thing at a time—the movement or exploring the colors and textures in the environment. If helpful, you can go into the environment with them and accompany them as they experience their environment.

- *A client is not able to find the right container or make a small container.* Stay beside the client and help them to explore the different containers available, and once they have decided on one, help them to explore potential materials to put on the container. Stay beside them while they are making this.

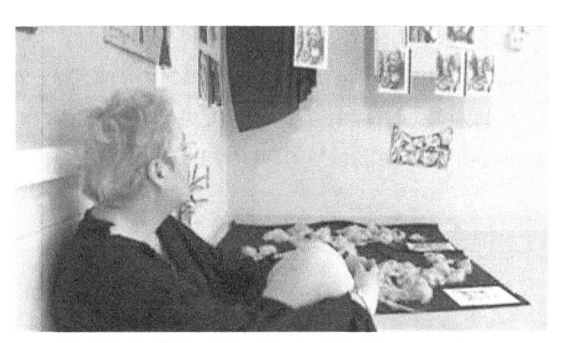

Gale Ostroff looking at *Environment*

My Process
Life-Size Environment Exercise

> It was an effortless process, everything came together easily, and I seemed to know exactly what I needed. The structure became a solid cave, and even though there are bones in the cave I want to go in to sing to the bones and bring them to life. This is my purpose…
>
> I like being her—La Loba—I trust her, know her, something powerful about the relationship of death and life…

Small-Size Environment Exercise
TITLE: *COMING ALIVE*

> I used a wooden basket. I wasn't sure about materials but gathered straw, luminescent green and yellow fabric, a wooden snake, and small tree branches. I placed straw so it covered almost all of the basket outside and inside and placed three rocks on the outside ledge of the basket.
>
> When I look at it now, I feel satisfied. The process was fun and quick. It felt obvious and not intricate, but large strokes, messy, almost as if the basket was the fire itself and the bones becoming alive. La Loba is not in it but somewhere behind, bringing it to life. When I look at it now it looks messy, disorganized, hard to know what's going on but also organic and alive. Something is happening, but hard to see exactly what it is.
>
> I want to enter and stay in the large environment; however, the small environment is self-contained: doesn't need me. There is a process happening all on its own and I have to trust…

CHAPTER 16

Directing Someone Else

She entered the room and then sat down slumped in a chair, not making eye contact and barely speaking. She spoke of her depression as if a curtain of darkness had descended and blocked out all the light. When we began our work together, she chose the character of the Greek goddess Persephone. In her embodiment of the role she always included heavy black material that she would drape around herself. During the session when she directed me as her character, I was crouched on the floor with the black material covering me like a shroud. She directed me to slowly push against the material as if I was trying to get out but could not. I did this and she watched. I asked if she wanted to make any changes to the movements and she said, "Do you think there is a way to get out?" And I responded, "Do you want to try another movement that you can teach me?" She said okay and draped the heavy black material over herself and crouched down low on the floor. As she tried different movements with the material, she lifted a corner of the material up with her hands and then a little more until she was able to see out. As she did this, she said, "I can let in a little light—not too much, just a little." Then she directed me to do the same movement and words. This time as she watched she had tears but also told me for the first time she felt some hope that her depression could lift. As she continued her work with Persephone through different creative mediums, she discovered that it was possible to descend into Hades (the dark underworld of the dead) but also re-emerge into the world of the living. When we ended our work, she was a different person—making eye contact, speaking with a clear voice, and walking with a sense of purpose. Now she felt her life was a quest, a hero's journey with profound challenges but also a sense of meaning. Her depression was no longer something shameful or hidden, but rather a badge of courage. She knew the depths of despair, but like Persephone, was able to find a way to move between the darkness and the light, and wanted to help others...

As opposed to verbal methods, in creative arts therapies, the experiential is central and multifaceted. It provides an arena where all kinds of behaviors, emotions, and attitudes can be expressed within a controlled and structured setting. In drama therapy, role play is a core aspect of the clinical sessions. Landy (1993) stresses the importance of identifying the client's internal cast of characters and bringing them out into the open. The goal is to increase the number of available roles in their repertoire so that they are not stuck in one or two destructive or ineffective roles. In his view, the ability to move from one role to another is a sign of health and social adeptness. Another approach to using role play, Developmental Transformations (DvT), is based on the psychoanalytic concept of free association and incorporates spontaneous playful improvisations between therapist and client (Johnson, 2009). In these sessions a multitude of diverse roles can be explored. In contrast, in psychodrama, specific scenes from real life are enacted by the group (Blatner, 1997). In all of these approaches, working with role play is the essential ingredient that allows for clients to gain perspective, insight, and ultimately transformation. One important aspect of working with role play is the option to either embody a role as the actor, or step back and be the director. This ability to negotiate between the two is an important therapeutic tool for negotiating aesthetic distance (see the sections on creative projection and aesthetic distance in Chapter 2). If a client is overwhelmed in a particular role, then they can gain distance by becoming the director, or in the opposite situation, they can gain more empathy by switching from director to actor.

At this stage in the *Story Within* process we have explored a variety of mediums and developed a deep connection with our character. Now it is important to gain some distance and perspective. For the first time instead of a personal creative exploration, we are being asked to direct someone else in the role of our character. We hand over our mask and costume and direct another person in specific choreography, sounds, and words. And then we step back and witness as our character comes to life on someone else. This process is often very intimate. After all, up until this point we were alone in our relationship with our character. We chose the story, character, and moment, made the mask, the costume, the soundscape, and the environment, and now we are handing this over to someone else and we are the witness. Once the other person puts on the character's mask, they are entering something very personal and perhaps something that has been kept hidden. Therefore, the exchange of characters must be done with tenderness and a deep respect for the significance of the process.

Finding the Movements, Sounds, and Words

Have your mask and costume available. You need enough space to do your initial movement exploration and teach someone else the movement.

Before you direct someone else you need to find a phrase of movement with words or sounds that clearly expresses your character in the moment you chose. It is essential to spend time with this aspect so that you explore different qualities of movements, sounds, and words, until you have a deep sense of knowing that it is right and complete. The movements should be simple enough to teach someone else and yet specific enough that they truly express your character. Once this is done you are ready to teach the movements, sounds, and words to someone else. Remember that you are the director and you can ask for what you want in terms of the exact quality of movement, the amount of tension, sense of weight, facial expression, and tone of voice. Of course, it will look different on another body and the person will bring their unique personality into the embodiment. This is actually what makes this experience so profound—the meeting of your specific choreography with the other person's interpretation and somatic expression. Now in addition to your own experience of your character, you have a new and fresh perspective. At this stage of the process this can be very illuminating and initiate a new level of understanding and insight.

FINDING THE CHARACTER'S MOVEMENTS, SOUNDS, AND WORDS EXERCISE

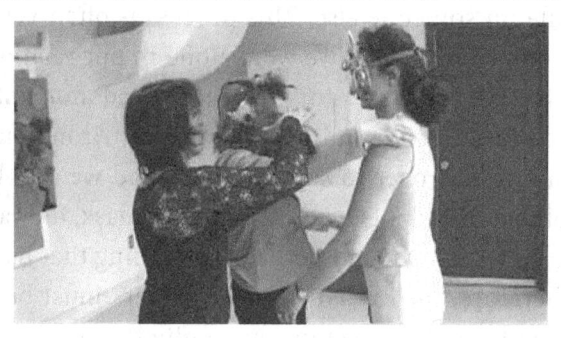

Kalie Rae Directing Two Others

1. Take some time to warm up your body, exploring different movement qualities such as (a) sense of weight (heavy, strong, light); (b) sense of body tension (tense or free flow); and (c) sense of direction (focussed and direct, or indirect, unfocussed). Then begin to feel your body and movements transform to embody your character.

2. Find a specific movement phrase or series of movements that expresses your character in the moment you chose. Try to make the movements as clear as possible and be able to repeat the exact movements over and over until you really know them. Experiment with different movement phrases and qualities of movement until you feel it is right.

3. Once you have the movement phrase you can add sounds or specific words that add to the expression. (Your sounds, words, and movements may all come at once, which is fine.) Again, be specific about the exact quality of the sounds and words in terms of volume, and emotion.

4. Once you have the movements, sounds, and words, try them with your mask and costume.

DIRECTING SOMEONE ELSE EXERCISE

1. Find a partner from your circle of support and teach them the movements, sounds, and words. Do not use the masks and costume until they have totally learned the embodiment the exact way you want it.

2. You are the director, so feel free to ask them to change the way they are doing the movements, the sounds, or the words to get the quality you want. Be kind and supportive to your partner and realize they have a different body and may not be able to physically enact exactly what you did. Find a way that they can accomplish a similar movement that expresses the quality you want.

3. Once they have the embodiment the way you want it, then have them try it with the mask and costume. Then give them any feedback regarding changes you might want and have them do it again. You may want to video them for your own personal records. (Obviously you will not make this public or show it to anyone else.)

4. When they have finished the embodiment, they must de-role, take off the mask and the costume, shake off their body, and let go of the character.

5. Ask the person how they felt in the role of your character. Without interpretation or analysis, have them tell you their own personal experience of how it felt in the role. For example, "I felt very ancient; the load I was carrying was heavy and hard to hold, but when I lifted my arms to the sky, I felt lighter as if something had fallen away. My arms were lighter and the sense of having to hold this load left…" It doesn't matter what they say as long as it is authentic to their direct experience. This is not an intellectual discussion, an interpretation, or analysis but rather a very personal response to a deeply intimate experience. Then you tell them how it felt to witness them, and you can continue to discuss the process. Stay with sharing your personal

experience rather than going into an intellectual discussion or analysis as this will take away from the experience.

6. Then switch roles so the other person has a chance to direct you in their character.

Working with Clients

If you are doing this individually with your client, have them direct you in the role of their character. You need to be willing to be vulnerable and allow yourself to try out different movements and sounds even if they are a bit uncomfortable. Obviously, if you cannot physically enact the movements or the sounds or words are truly offensive to you, you may have to modify, but try as much as possible to do their exact movements, sounds, and words. This will be an interesting experience in terms of the power differential and the therapeutic relationship as they are now in charge. You are always the therapist and are doing this embodiment in service of their process. However, it does involve a role reversal in terms of them being the director and you in a more vulnerable position of trying to do their movements. This can be very empowering for your client and demonstrate your trust in their process and their ability to direct you. Often this leads to an even more profound therapeutic alliance and connection. This exercise also gives clients an opportunity to direct the other person exactly how they want them to be in terms of quality of movement, sounds, and expression. They also hear the feedback of the person playing the role of their character. Hearing personal feedback about how it feels for another person to be in the role of their character is often illuminating.

Things to Watch Out For

- *The client cannot find a movement expression for their character.* Help them in the movement exploration and move with them so they don't feel so self-conscious or alone. As you move with them, explore different movement qualities and sounds and words. Help them to identify what feels most connected to their character. You can also have them teach one posture or one small movement that feels right, and they can just witness that and go back and forth, with them finding a posture or movement and teaching you until they feel more confident.

- *The client cannot give you direction.* Help them by asking questions about the quality of movement, expression, sounds, words, etc. Keep asking and encouraging them to give you more explicit directions. For someone who has difficulty with decisions, or has low self-esteem, or who has never had the opportunity to state what they want, this can be a real challenge, but also, once accomplished, very empowering.

- *The client becomes overwhelmed when finding a movement.* Help them by immediately asking them to stop and take a break and then teach you one aspect of the movement, for example a small hand gesture, or whatever feels the least emotional. They teach you this one aspect of movement and then stay in the role of witness and director until they become more comfortable.

My Process
Finding the Character's Movements, Sounds, and Words Exercise

> It took a little while to get it exactly right and changed every time. At the beginning it felt so heavy and burdensome but transformed into something powerful, primal, and a bit scary when La Loba was creating life. First couple of times I ended with a high singing note, but the last time just ended naturally and quietly standing with my hands cupping my mouth and breathing out. Interesting that the weight changed from heavy to light and ended with air. I need to let go of carrying the bones…

Afterwards I felt very emotional, tears came, exhausted, as if my body worked through something…

Directing Someone Else Exercise

Feedback from the person embodying my character: "In the beginning a sense of a burden, aging, heavy, and then excitement of finding the right bones, building to a final release as if smoke is coming out of all parts of me. The last part feels as if I'm seeing what has been created out of the dust, bones, out of smoke, and sending it off into the world with love…"

My Reaction

In all my years of working with this approach I've never done this part—never asked anyone else to embody my character.

So powerful to see her do this. It made me realize how much I like and am in awe of La Loba—her strength, her determination, her power, and her ability to create life. I didn't see it as a creation myth of birthing until I saw La Loba embodied in someone else and received her feedback…

Still not sure what La Loba is teaching me…but I am in awe of her certainty, clarity about what bones she should gather, which ones will be able to come to life. Does it matter which bones? Could any of them come to life? What gives her the power, the bones themselves, the song, the fire, the whole process? She is separate from her creation, from the wolf—she watches it go—with love—with awe—with connection. It is at the same time part of her and separate. Is this my relationship with my creations—my films, this book?

CHAPTER 17

Obstacle and Helper

I walked through the hallway that smelled strongly of disinfectant and urine, waving to the elderly women parked along the sides in their wheelchairs. This was my first professional job as a creative arts therapist in a "nursing home" and I led groups where we sang, moved with scarves, and participants told stories about their lives. Today I was asked to see a woman who was dying of cancer, bedridden, and refused any therapy or social interaction. As I entered her room she looked up from the bed and grabbed the magazine she was reading and threw it at me, yelling, "I don't need any of your god-damn feel-good bullshit!" I ducked and retreated into the doorway. Stunned and not sure what to do, I left and went back to see my supervisor stating that there was no way I could do therapy with this woman. The wise head nurse looked at me kindly and said, "She is suffering and angry and if you go back and find a way to reach her, she will end up being your greatest teacher." Reluctantly, I went back into the room. This time the woman said "Oh, not you again!" and proceeded to ignore me. She read magazines and I decided I would read stories out loud whether she was listening or not. I went to see her every day and she continued to ignore me, and I continued to read stories. One day I read the story of Scheherazade, about a king who, because his first wife betrayed him, marries and then beheads a different woman each day. Scheherazade agreed to marry the King and tells him a new story every night. The King is so intrigued he saves her life. When I finished reading, my uninterested patient, lying on her bed, looked up at me for the first time, laughed bitterly, and said, "I understand the King—everyone betrays you—might as well just behead them…" I suggested she might want to work with that character and surprisingly she said, "Why not?" After a few weeks I asked her to find the Obstacle and the

> Helper in the story. Immediately she chose Scheherazade as the Helper and the King's fear of betrayal as the Obstacle. We made masks for both and she directed me to embody each one and how her character, the King, would interact with them. At one point as she directed me as the "fear of betrayal" to crouch down and hide beneath a chair, she became very angry and then sad. She told me her parents had betrayed her by getting divorced and then leaving her with an aunt who neglected and abused her as a child. So she had lived her life in anger. However, she had a sister who she had loved as a child but rarely spoke to now. After the session I asked if she might want to contact her sister. She did and the sister came to visit. A month later the woman died, but for the last month of her life she laughed and cried with her sister, apologized, and connected with the nurses and a few of the other patients. She proudly asked to have her masks hung up in her room, and one of the last things she said to me was "Scheherazade saved me..."

Every story has an Obstacle, something that challenges the protagonist and tries to keep them from reaching their goal. Usually there is also a Helper, some guiding force, whether animate or inanimate, that supports the hero's quest or destiny. The purpose of the quest is different for each story. It can be to retrieve a loved one, attain knowledge, complete a task, or face inner demons. However, there is always a rite of passage, some challenge that is necessary to get through. And in the process of discovering how to deal with inner or outer demons and monsters or how to get by the guardians of the treasure, the protagonist learns something essential about themselves. Thus, the story itself is the teacher, just as the stories of Scheherazade saved her life, and ultimately all the women in the kingdom since the King himself was healed. And it was the story that saved my dying patient in the nursing home. She still had cancer and she still died; however, the story helped her find a way to heal her childhood trauma so that in the last days of her life she found love.

At this stage of the process in the *Story Within*, we have a strong identification with our character and have been immersed with making masks, movements, environments, and sounds, and even witnessing our character and mask on someone else. Gradually, and over time, we have entered a mythic world where the unconscious and conscious meet and the symbolic world connects in some mysterious way to our daily life. Now we must go even deeper into our story and identify what the obstacle and helper are, even though from a purely narrative and linear perspective it may seem obvious that the monster or villain is the Obstacle. However, the *Story Within* process is not about the narrative structure of the story, but rather the personal relationship between us and our character. This relationship is what matters, and even though two people may choose the same character, their Obstacle and Helper may be vastly different. For example, in the traditional Inuit story of Sedna, the Sea Goddess, there is a chilling moment when during a storm Sedna is holding on to the side of the boat with her hands, and to save himself and the boat, her father chops off her fingers. For one of my clients this moment was the Obstacle and led them to discover a hidden trauma in their own life. While for another client this same moment in the story was the Helper—the cutting off of the fingers was a necessary separation that Sedna and this client needed to face. So as we search for the Obstacle and Helper it is important to let ourselves be surprised and have the answer emerge through our intuition or unconscious. What our logical minds might think of as an obvious Helper, such as a fairy godmother, a prince, good witch Glinda, or Gandalf, may turn out to be the Obstacle. It really depends on where the story is trying to lead us, and we won't know that until the end of the process. It takes great courage to trust the unknown, to have faith in this mysterious journey with our character, and to be willing to go to places we have never been before.

FINDING THE OBSTACLE AND HELPER EXERCISE

Preparation
You need enough space to move in and to create a scene with two other people.

Materials
You need to have your mask and costume and art materials, fabrics, objects, etc. to create masks and/or objects to represent the Obstacle and Helper.

Finding the Obstacle and Helper

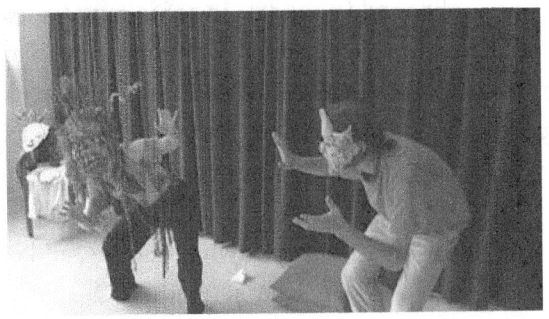

Obstacle and Helper by Benedicte Deschamps

1. Look through your story, particularly the moment that you chose, and identify a character or a part of the narrative that feels like the Obstacle. Trust your intuition and what comes up organically rather than using your rational mind or analysis. It can be a specific character or element in the story, or something abstract such as "the King's fear of betrayal." Let yourself be surprised.

2. Go through the same process for the Helper.

3. Once both the Obstacle and the Helper are clearly identified, begin to work creatively with each one.

4. First embody your character and the task it wants to accomplish or what it wants to do and begin to imagine how the Obstacle tries to stop your character and how the Helper tries to assist.

5. Find a movement and sounds/words that express the Obstacle and how it interacts with your character. Once you find the right movements and sounds/words, do it several times until you know it well.

6. Go through the same process for the Helper.

7. Once you have the movements/sounds/words for both the Obstacle and the Helper, then create or find objects that represent each one. It could be that you make a mask for the Obstacle and another mask for the Helper. Or you make a mask for the Obstacle and have fabric and an object that represent

the Helper. What is important is that you have something tangible and outside yourself that can be worn by someone else.

8. Spend some time embodying the Obstacle with the movements/sounds/words and mask/object costume and then do the same for the Helper.

Obstacle and Helper Scene Embodied

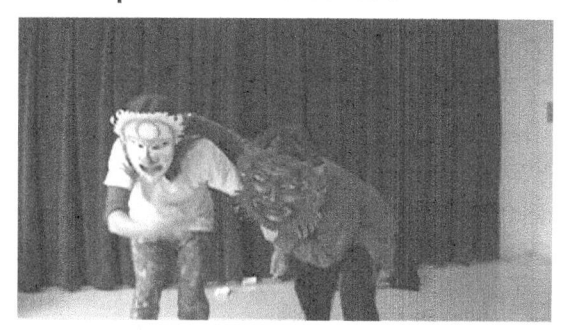

Obstacle and Helper by David Jan

This can be a very emotional and vulnerable process, so please only work with those who you trust will take it seriously. If at any time it feels too overwhelming, stop, take a break, or find additional support.

1. You may want to set up the space so that you have objects, fabric, or "environments" for the scene to take place. Do this before you start working together.

2. Partner up with two other people from your circle of support and tell them about the Obstacle and Helper and then teach them the movements/sounds/words and how each one will interact with your character.

3. Watch them do the movements/sounds/words and make sure they get it exactly how you want it in terms of movement, voice quality, and expression.

4. Then have them put on the masks/costumes/fabric/objects and witness them embodying the Obstacle and Helper.

5. Give them any feedback necessary so that it is exactly how you want it.

6. Then put on your character's mask and costume and you embody your character trying to do what it wants to do in the moment you chose, and the other two people will embody the Obstacle and Helper interacting with you as your character. All three of you will be embodying your roles.

7. Once you have embodied your character's interaction with its Obstacle and Helper, if it didn't feel quite right give the other two people feedback so that they can make the necessary changes and try the process again.

8. Once the embodiment feels right, everyone de-roles (takes off the mask, costume, etc.) and the person who played the Obstacle tells you how they felt in the role and how it was to interact with your character and the Helper. Then the person who played the Helper tells you how they felt in the role interacting with your character and with the Obstacle.

9. Then switch roles so someone else takes a turn directing their Obstacle and Helper.

10. Continue to discuss the process but stay with what happened and feelings that emerged rather than interpretation or analysis.

Working with Clients

For clients in a well-functioning group, or even a group that is struggling but sincere in its efforts, the process of working together in this exercise can be profound. For the client who is sharing and then directing others as their Obstacle and Helper, it can be both very vulnerable and very healing. Perhaps for the first time they have others willing to share their pain and inner struggles. And for the group members who are embodying someone's Obstacle and Helper it can be very moving to be trusted with this responsibility of entering a role that is so intimate and personal. Often sharing this process together brings group members closer and can bring them from one stage of the group process to the next stage.

Obstacle

When clients choose the Obstacle, it becomes something outside of themselves that they can work with as an object. This makes it tangible and they can direct how the Obstacle interacts with their character. The Obstacle can be surprising (when something genuinely surprises your clients, you know they have fully entered the unconscious and they are following rather than leading). In a supportive, well-functioning group, another person can play the Obstacle, or you can take on that role if in individual therapy.

Helper

It is important for clients to know there is always a Helper, even if inanimate or unseen. For many clients who have experienced trauma or abuse, it can be difficult to accept help, or trust that help is available. The process of finding and working with a Helper in the story can be transformative as they learn they can ask for help and receive it. In a supportive, well-functioning group, another person can play the Helper, or you can take on that role if in individual therapy.

Things to Watch Out For

- *Clients are not able to identify the Obstacle and/or Helper in their story.* You can work with them by going over the elements in the story, asking them to let you know their emotional responses. For some clients it may be helpful to ask them to do a brief creative expression through any medium of what they see as potential Obstacles and Helpers around the moment they chose. Working creatively may help to allow the unconscious to come through and guide them to what is most poignant. You can also encourage them to trust whatever comes up even if it does not make sense.

- *Others in the group are not willing or able to embody the Obstacle and Helper.* This can happen in groups that are more insecure and unstable. If so, you need to intervene more and give more explicit guidelines about why the role of embodying is so crucial, that they are in service of the one who is directing, and that if they feel the movement of the role is too difficult they can switch partners and find something they feel they can do. Encouraging all group members to embrace some discomfort as a necessary part of growth can normalize the anxiety and give a sense of meaning to their discomfort.

- *Group members give inappropriate feedback to the director.* Some group members may try and interpret or make judgments on the role they embodied. It is essential that this be discouraged and they be reminded that they only share their personal feelings playing the role using "I" statements. The feedback aspect of all the group exercises is a crucial component of the process and all the group members become an integral part of each other's character and story.

My Process
Obstacle
"She collects and preserves especially that which is in danger of being lost to the world…"

Helper
"The wolf creature begins to breathe."

My Response to Finding the Obstacle and Helper

> *The bones are lost to the world*
> *And I must find them*
> *Each one*
> *If I miss any—I am condemned…*
> *And yet I hear the wolf song*
> *Calling…head thrown back,*
> *Howling, laughing…*
> *I stand alone.*
> *No one can see me*
> *as my breath becomes life.*

I wasn't sure at first but knew the Obstacle had something to do with the bones and the Helper had something to do with the singing over the bones. When I read these words, I had a visceral reaction: "The bones being lost to the world" brought such great sadness that even now I still feel it…

Not sure why, but this is the most emotional. I feel vulnerable. How can I abandon the lost bones…the dead…those that need me to find them and carry them? And yet I long to sing, to breathe new life.

Obstacle and Helper Scene Embodied

I directed the Obstacle to seduce and drag me back to collect more bones, saying, "This one will be lost forever…unless you collect it now…"

Helper is trying to push me towards the fire, the singing, away from the collecting of bones; she says, "The wolf creature begins to breathe…"

In the scene it was very hard to leave the bones—as if I had to physically tear myself away from them. Felt responsible as if I was the only one who could save them—felt sad at leaving them. But hearing the soft howling and breath of the wolf allowed me to realize there was another choice…

Feedback from Person Playing the Obstacle

As the Obstacle there was an urgency, the phrases "lost forever" and "collect it now"—each time you slipped away I felt I would lose you—you would be lost to me—it was painful for me—I needed to seduce you to stay with the bones forever…

Feedback from Person Playing the Helper

As the wolf creature I felt that you were getting lost, made me want to howl at the moon and wake you up—give you breath—breathe into you with you… I wanted you to move forward…

CHAPTER 18

The Edge

I first saw her sitting in the hallway of the hospital, hair disheveled, pants torn and dirty, posture slumped, and yet totally engrossed in the book she was reading. I had been warned that this homeless adolescent, who often ended up in the emergency room beaten and filled with drugs, would not come to sessions. However, the fact that she cared enough about reading to somehow find and keep a book made me hopeful. She entered the room wary and only looked up when I asked her to tell me what the book was about. She said, "You really want to know?" I said, "Yes." She described the characters in detail and said there was a surprise ending. I asked if I could borrow the book and we could talk about it next time. She looked suspicious and asked if this was some sort of trick to get her to come back. I smiled and told her that I promised to read the book. She did show up for the next session and we discussed the book and then I asked if she liked fairy tales or myths and we looked through books together. When I read some titles out loud to her, she pointed to "The Handless Maiden" without even reading it. This is a story about a girl whose father had inadvertently given her to the devil and to save himself chops off his daughter's hands. The daughter flees into the forest where she gradually grows new hands. We read it together and then she began to work with it. However, instead of going through all the steps, she spent every session making hands out of clay, out of wire, out of fabric, out of anything she could find. For months she showed up and without a word spent the session making hands. I knew enough not to interrupt her or try to make her talk. If I had she would have bolted and never returned. Both of us trusted that what she was doing was important even if neither of us knew what it was. After several months, during one session I brought some rope into the room. As she was making hands out of clay she saw the rope and quickly grabbed it and tied the rope tightly around each hand, attaching the hands to a chair. Then she stood back, looked at it and froze. Her body started shaking uncontrollably and she was gasping for breath. I came close but didn't touch her. Then she broke down and started sobbing. I sat beside her. Gradually she told me her story. When she was a very young girl, around age five or six, her father tied her hands to the bed and raped her. This continued for several years until she ran away around age ten. She was in a foster home and then by age 12 was living on the streets. I realized that her unconscious had led her to the story of "The Handless Maiden" and that the making of hands was the beginning of her healing. When she saw the rope tied around the hands, that was her "Edge" and took her right back to the experience of her early abuse and trauma. After this session we worked on her reclaiming her own hands following the journey of "The Handless Maiden." Instead of making hands out of clay she began moving her own hands through space and letting her hands reach out for materials, for things in the room, and eventually for me. By the last session she was living in a group home and went back to high school. She told me she wanted to work with homeless youth. She asked me why I had believed in her and I said, "Because I could see you liked stories." And she smiled and said, "Yeah, that's why I thought you might not be so bad either."

We all carry a place deep inside of us that is scary or so uncomfortable that we will do anything to avoid it. For the girl in the above story it was a memory of the extreme sexual abuse and trauma she suffered as a young child. For many of us our hidden stories are not so brutal; however, they can still unconsciously control how we perceive ourselves and others. For example, in elementary and junior high I was the victim of anti-Semitism. I was called "a Dirty Jew" on my first day of school, and watched boys in class laugh at photos of gas chambers and concentration camps. I remember being on the doorstep of one of my classmate's homes with the only person of color in the class and the mother opening the door and telling us very politely that she was sorry, but we could not enter her house. As we walked away, I noticed a confederate flag flying in the front yard. As a child I felt helpless, ashamed, and that somehow I was at "fault" for being different. School became a place of trauma and I acted out in class, and did poorly, labeled a "bad girl." Until recently these memories stayed hidden and buried deep in my unconscious. As an adult I remembered that it happened, but in my own personal therapy I never mentioned it. During the writing of this book, as you know, I followed the steps of the *Story Within*, working with the character of La Loba, Wolf Woman. She lives alone and collects bones that would be lost to the world and sings over them, bringing them to life. In working with this story and facing my "Edge," I realized the bones were those hidden childhood memories and how they affected the way I see myself even now, so many years later. As I write these words, tears form, the emotions are still raw, the insights still fresh, and yet something deep within has also released and healed, and I am so grateful to La Loba. Each one of us has a different "Edge" and it takes courage and preparation to be able to face it. We, who have ventured on this mythic path, entering the world of our character, exploring our creative voice, have unconsciously and gradually prepared for this most difficult and yet essential step. Even though the Edge we create is for our character, it can lead us directly to our own fears and inner hidden story.

The word "edge" has different meanings. It can be the outside limit of an object, area, or surface, the border, or the sharpened side of a blade or weapon. As a verb it implies moving gradually, carefully, to advance slowly. All these meanings are applicable for the way the "Edge" is used in the *Story Within* process. When we face a hidden and potentially traumatic part of ourselves, we need to approach it gradually and over time so that we feel safe and prepared. The idea of the Edge is that it is a place we want to avoid and is deeply uncomfortable; however, it is also a place that we are now ready to face. The goal is not to go over the Edge and fall apart, but through our character and all the previous work find the courage to approach that which seemed unapproachable. It is also something that feels sharp and incisive like a blade that cuts through layers of our psyche to uncover what has been hidden and inaccessible. This step in the

Story Within process is the one that brings us closer to understanding why this story and character chose us and what it was trying to lead us to face in ourselves. We are asked to create something that symbolizes our "scary or uncomfortable interior place" or Edge, using any artistic media (art materials, fabric, furniture, whatever inspires us). Once this has been made, we physically move toward the art work object, first while taking on the role of our character, and secondly as ourselves out of character. Often, we notice that our character approaches the Edge in a very different manner than we do. This process often solidifies the commonalities and differences between the character and ourselves and makes us begin to examine the uncomfortable place inside us in a new way. It has now been expressed as something external that is concrete, and therefore not as terrifying. It may even, surprisingly, be perceived as something treasured or beautiful. This also sets up the beginning of a separation from our character.

THE EDGE EXERCISE

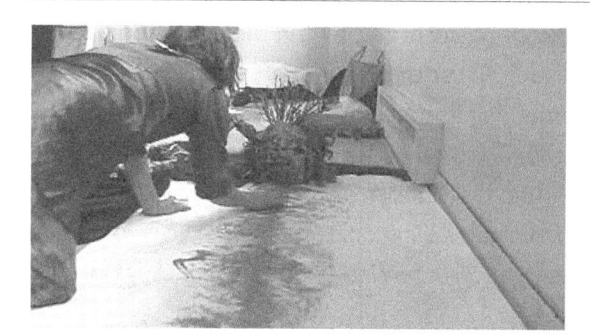

Edge by Benedicte Deschamps

This exercise can elicit strong emotions. Please use your circle as support or seek additional professional help if needed.

Preparation

You need space to create something outside yourself and to be able to move around what you create.

Materials

You will need to have materials around the room that you can use for your creation, such as fabrics, wire, paper, cotton, rocks, chairs, tables, goggles, costumes, paint; the list is endless. Use what you have and let your imagination run wild!

The Exercise

1. Spend some time feeling your character and, as your character, walk around the room and begin to focus on the idea of an Edge. This is the place your character does not want to go to. You may also find that you are identifying the Edge in yourself and the uncomfortable feelings you avoid. It is fine for this exercise that the line between your character and you are blurred and the notion of what the Edge is can be vague and unclear, but the impetus is to create something that expresses this Edge.

2. Begin to gather materials, objects, whatever calls out to you. Let yourself be surprised by the materials and even by what you are creating. Trust that your character is now ready to show you something important. As you gather the materials, begin to shape them into some form that expresses this Edge, this place of profound discomfort. You can use chairs and tables, hang things from the ceiling or over shelves. Use your imagination to find the right structure to express the feelings of this Edge.

3. Continue using the materials, finalizing the form and structure of the expression. You do not need to have any idea or understanding of what it all means, just trust that whatever you have created is right and necessary.

4. Once the creation feels complete, walk away from it and look at it. Without interpretation or analysis, write in your journal what you see. Try as much as possible to stay with exactly what is present, such as the materials, the colors, the structure, the objects, the size, etc. And notice how you feel when you look

at it. What stands out? What surprises you? What emotions come up?

5. Then put away your journal and put on the mask and costume of your character. Spend a few moments embodying your character and then approach your Edge creation as your character. Let your character approach it, interact with it, make sounds, speak, move, in whatever way feels authentic for your character. It could be that your character tries to avoid this place, fights it, or tenderly caresses it. It doesn't matter what it looks like, only that it is authentic for your character.

6. Next take off the mask and costume and now approach the Edge creation as yourself. Let yourself approach it, interact with it, make sounds, speak, move, in whatever way feels authentic to you. If you don't want to approach it, find a way to relate to it from far away. Or perhaps you want to be close and choose to lie down right in the center. It doesn't matter what it looks like, only that it is authentic for you.

7. Return to your mask and costume and put them on again and approach the Edge as your character. You may find your character interacts a bit differently this time. Trust that whatever happens is okay and important.

8. Finally, take off your mask and costume and for the last time approach it again as yourself. You may find that you interact a bit differently this time. Trust that whatever happens is okay and important.

9. Take some time to reflect on what happened and write in your journal. This is often when connections become clear between your chosen story and character and your own personal life and hidden stories. Let whatever insights or discoveries have emerged to be honored and described in whatever language feels right for now. If it is helpful you can use other mediums to express these discoveries (art, music, movement, drama). This exercise and reflection can often bring up strong emotions,

so be gentle with yourself and, if necessary, ask for support from your witness(es). Let yourself cry, laugh, sigh, or lie down, whatever comes up organically.

10. When you are ready, come together with your witness(es) and share what you choose to with them. It may feel too soon to share, and if so, just share your creation with them describing whatever aspects of it you want. As you describe your creation you may spontaneously begin to share some of your insights and discoveries with your witness(es).

11. Your witness's job is to be a supportive presence, holding space for you as you share your experience. This is often a very vulnerable time, and whatever insights or discoveries have emerged, they are fragile and raw. Therefore, it is important that the witness reflect what you have shared and do not give their own interpretations or analysis. They are there to support what came up for you in terms of your own Edge and personal connections between your story and your own life.

12. When you are finished sharing with your witness, thank them and then take a photo of your Edge creation. Then decide what you want to do with it. Based on space limitation you may have to take it down. If so, find a ritual way of thanking it and then taking it apart. Or, if possible, and it feels right, leave it up for as long as you want, maybe even visiting it over the next week.

13. This exercise is often one of the most demanding emotionally, so please be gentle with yourself and take it easy. If possible, rest after completing this exercise and nourish yourself with good food, sleep, and whatever replenishes your spirit.

Working with Clients

In this exercise, clients are creating something outside of themselves that expresses a deeply uncomfortable place. Even though it is still in the context of the character and story, it is bringing them close to their own personal Edge. Everyone has a different Edge.

By creatively expressing these deeply uncomfortable feelings onto something concrete and outside themselves, they can gain insight and perspective. This is the time in the process when the drama–life connections become apparent and the reason for why the client chose the story is revealed.

As therapists it is important to recognize where our own personal Edge is. We cannot go anywhere with those we work with unless we have explored these areas within ourselves. If our own hidden stories and internal Edge have to do with shame, we may try and avoid this with our clients. Not that we won't address it, but we may find ourselves trying to "rescue" or make it "better" rather than sitting with the client in their discomfort. When we as therapists are willing to explore through working with story, character, and creativity, our own inner wounds, we become much more profound therapists.

Things to Watch Out For

- *Clients cannot create an Edge.* Help them by working alongside and suggesting they try a variety of materials, seeing how each one feels. You can even build the creative structure with them, always questioning and taking directions from them. It can be an overwhelming task, and having you working with them allows for more safety.

- *Clients become overwhelmed either as their character or as themselves.* Help them by stepping in and having them direct you as their character or as themselves. This way they can gain some distance and perspective yet continue with the exercise. If this is still overwhelming, then you can use the Edge creation as an object without the embodiment aspects that you and your client can look at and discuss together.

- *Clients are not able to separate character and self.* Sometimes the identification and projection onto the character is so strong that the separation process is difficult. Help them by encouraging them to de-role after embodying their character and make a distinction between their character and themselves.

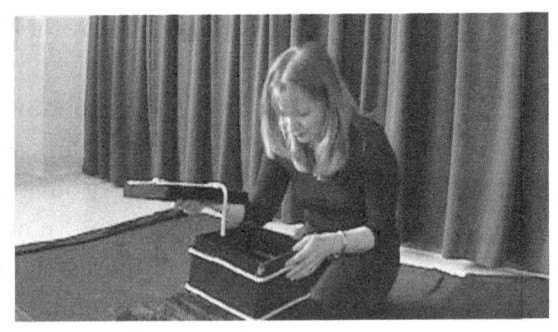

Edge by Patti Dray

My Process
The Edge Creation

I used brown fabric splashed with red paint, wire, skeletal masks, and black thick hose. I took a blue painted blank mask and ripped it (very satisfying) and hung it in a wooden picture frame and put this in the front of the creation. Then I put flowers over the skeletal masks. Lastly, I found a mirror and put it in the very back of my Edge.

When I look at it, I feel sad. Do all things lead to the mirror? I can't see myself—too much stuff in the way, it's like everything before the mirror is a distraction, an illusion, a trap. The fragmented blue mask on the frame—is this how I see myself? Fragmented? No substance? Hanging suspended…?

Embodiment
As Character

La Loba was not afraid, approached and honored each mask, and fed them with rocks and sang an ancient chant. Then she shook the rocks, went over to the mirror, and looked at herself as La Loba—curious, fierce, strong, solid…

As Myself

This was much harder, I didn't want to go near it, circled around the outside, then I looked at each skeletal mask and it became clear what each one was: the childhood anti-Semitism, the disconnect from myself, deaths of my brother, my best friend, when they were way too young… The fragmented mask in the front is how I see myself. Finally, I picked up the mirror and looked at myself first from arm's length, then brought the mirror closer and really looked, saw my tired eyes and had compassion for myself, then brought the mirror closer and kissed my image—this brought sobs from deep inside…

I see myself as fragmented not whole, tried so hard to be "good." I was controlled by the "bones," the old masks, couldn't see my own beauty, my own wholeness, wisdom, intelligence, creativity. Who am I without my masks? I just realized that La Loba is creating herself anew when she brings the bones to life. She is the bones, the wolf, the old woman and the young woman laughing…

CHAPTER 19

Final Presentation/Ritual

My Process

I set up three sculptures each with masks, representing La Loba, the Wolf, and the Edge. Working with my circle of support I had each person take two rocks. Then I asked them to hold them and make a noise with them as we walked together toward the sculptures. I started singing and chanting, letting the primal sounds come through me…it felt organic and powerful, as if La Loba was singing to the bones…

Then I introduced my circle of support to the sculpture of La Loba and said, "I was initially drawn to the bones but did not know why. La Loba is strong, ancient, powerful, and for her the bones were not a burden, she knew that she would breathe life into them… but I didn't know that. For me the bones felt like a heavy burden…" Then I introduced the Wolf as my Helper. And finally, I gathered my circle around my Edge sculpture and picked up the skeletal masks and introduced the "bones," the anti-Semitism I experienced as a child, being alone on the playground, not understanding why it was happening… For all these years this was hidden, buried, shameful… As I shared all this I cried, and yet felt held by the circle…

Responses from My Circle of Support

- "The bones are what is left after someone dies, they remain… and you needed to go to the core, to the bones…"

- "I was struck by you being alone on the playground, and not understanding why, but now you have new understanding and compassion…"
- "Now you are bringing the bones out into the world."
- "What you experienced as a child has made you who you are."

I needed to do this step, needed to uncover the bones and have them be seen by others and loved. Now I feel such tenderness for my Edge, for what was hidden and secret… La Loba gives me courage to not only face my own wounds but to bring them out into the world…to trust that by sharing them I am opening the door for others…

Student Final Presentations/Rituals

- She was Cassandra and had us lie on the floor as she played a recorded soundscape she had created. She asked us to close our eyes and we were transported to an ancient time…
- He was Alice in Wonderland, and as we held up a giant mirror and gave him encouragement, he walked through…
- She was Persephone and we all entered the dark room one at a time and she welcomed us to Hades…
- He was Kai from "The Snow Queen" and his mask shattered on the floor into tiny pieces that he had us collect one by one…
- She was Sedna, and her paintings of her bloody hands and the beauty and peace of the ocean were placed on the wall and on the floor and she asked us to take time with each one…
- She was the witch in "Hansel and Gretel" and made a multi-layered cake that she offered to each one of us as she told her story…
- He was Atalanta and made an animated video of his character running away…

- She was the woman from "The Woman and the Bear," and she made a giant soft sculpture of a bear, and to the sound of throat singing we all danced in front of the bear...

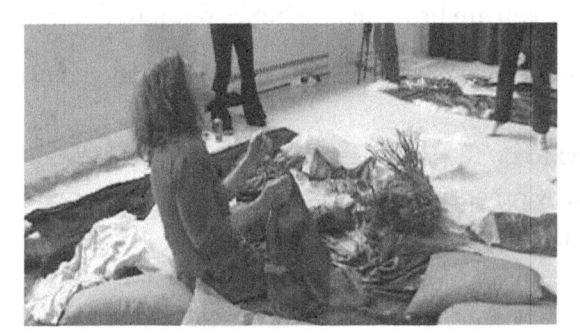

Final Ritual by Benedicte Deschamps

The last step in the *Story Within* process is to present a creative expression of our personal journey with our character. This can be in the form of a performance, painting, sculpture, video, poem, story, audio recording, song, mixed media, or any artistic medium. From the first exercise, *Encounter*, we have been exploring our creativity and creative projection, allowing our intuition and story itself to lead us. We worked hard to let go of interpretation and analysis so that we could truly discover something new. Now is the time when we look over everything we have done, all our creations, responses, masks, and embodiment, and notice the patterns and recurrent themes. We may find that the seeds for our journey were planted right in the first two exercises; our unconscious and the artistic mediums themselves were ready and waiting to guide us. Once we found our story and character then we could enter a mythic landscape and be held by something larger, archetypal. Within our story was a hidden treasure that at first was elusive and mysterious and only gradually revealed itself. At each step we were faced with challenges, with doubt, with misgiving about why we were engaged in such a strange process. But something compelled us to continue, to trust that our character would help us to be able to uncover something buried deep within. All the previous steps prepared us to face our Edge. We created and embodied our mask, we directed others, we identified the Obstacle and Helper, and we learned to trust our intuition to guide us. All of this took great courage and fortitude and now we are ready to make the connection between our character and our own life. Now we can analyze and interpret what this journey has been about. However, to do that we need to examine everything that has come before and find a creative way to synthesize what we have learned. It is not enough to understand cognitively; we must integrate it through a creative expression. And our creation must be witnessed.

As we move through the steps of the *Story Within*, we are also moving through the stages of creative process. We began in the preparation stage and then became immersed in exploring artistic mediums. After a while we needed a break from all of it to incubate. Then, if we were fortunate, insights happened and some part of us became illuminated. Now in this last step we are entering the validation stage where we take our insights and everything we have learned into the real world. Therefore, it is essential that your *Final Presentation/Ritual* is seen and heard by others. It should be your circle of support, or your therapist if doing this in therapy. Additionally, you could invite trusted friends, family, or anyone that you feel will be supportive and can hold the space. Not only are we witnessed but we determine exactly how we want to be seen or heard. We decide the role, placement, and response of our witnesses. This opportunity to be able to ask for how we want to be seen can in itself be healing. The *Final Presentation/Ritual* provides closure with our character, a creative way to separate and honor all of what our story and character taught us.

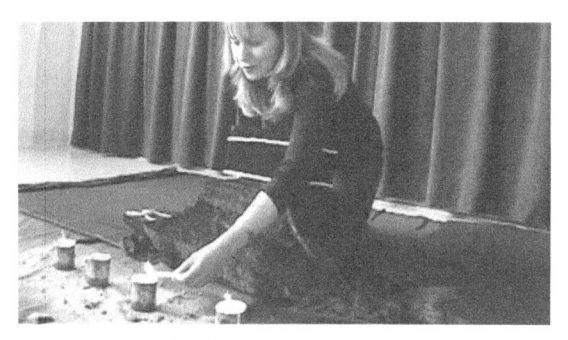

Final Ritual by Patty Dray

FINAL PRESENTATION/RITUAL

Preparation

You will need to determine the space, the format, the necessary materials, and role of your witnesses.

Materials

1. Look over all your creations (photos of artistic creations, audio recordings of soundscape, written work, everything in your journal) from the beginning of the process.

2. Once you have all your materials, notice what mediums you used and if there are patterns in terms of colors, mediums, shapes, movements, textures, sounds, etc.

3. Which mediums were rewarding? Which mediums were challenging? Which mediums led to new insights? Which mediums disappointed you? Which mediums surprised you?

4. Analyze your creative DNA. What is your primary perception—visual, auditory, tactile, kinesthetic, emotional, conceptual, taste, smell? (Review the discussion of creative DNA in Chapter 3 for more details.) What is your most utilized perception, the way you normally experience the world? Which perception moves you the most? Which perception is recuperative? Which perception do you experience the least? (Look over your answers from the questionnaire in Chapter 3 and notice if the responses are the same.)

5. How did you go through the stages of creative process? When were you in each stage?

Working with Your Story and Character

1. What was the process of choosing your story, character, and moment?

2. How did working with different mediums affect your relationship with your character? Which mediums brought you closer, or

farther away? Which mediums were transitional, transformative, or frightening?

3. What did the story and character teach you? Where did it lead? What was the *story* of your relationship with your character?

4. What specific exercises were most important and crucial in your journey? What were the patterns and themes that emerged along the way? What were the transitional moments?

5. What was your experience of being witnessed (and being a witness if this is applicable)?

6. What was your experience of working with your circle of support? Or with your therapist in the context of personal therapy?

The Exercise

1. Once you have looked over everything and done your analysis, then you begin to decide on your *Final Presentation/Ritual*. It should be an original creative expression, through whatever creative medium(s) you choose, of the story of your *personal* relationship with your character from the beginning to where you are now in the relationship. You can include a brief outline of your story, but the goal of this step is your own original creation.

2. The *Final Presentation/Ritual* should represent the key elements of your creative process throughout the course. You need to look over your own creative process to come up with a synthesis of this process expressed through the arts.

3. The *Final Presentation/Ritual* needs to be an original creative piece (performance, art work, sound recording, creative ritual with your witnesses). This is not a didactic presentation but a carefully constructed creative piece. You should create the presentation, but you can use members of your circle of support to help with technology, set up, or be part of it.

4. The more you work on preparing the *Final Presentation/Ritual*, the more powerful it will be for your process. It is extremely helpful to carefully construct the structure and format and have a clear beginning, middle, and end with attention to details. Try and pay attention to what medium(s) you will use, where in the room you will present, where your audience/witnesses will be, and how they are placed (sitting in a circle, standing in a line, lying on the floor, eyes open or closed, etc.).

5. Reflect on and consider carefully the role, placement, and response you want from your witnesses. How do you want them to respond, through what mediums and in what manner? Do you want them to be silent, to say something, to respond through art or movement? Be specific and tell them beforehand.

6. Your circle of support have been witnesses and taken part in your journey. This presentation is part of your closure with the group (if applicable).

7. The preparation for the final presentation is the time to make the character/life connections. What has come up for you? What has your character taught you? What has the journey been like? What were the surprises, the challenges, the insights, the hidden treasures, the question marks, and the confusions? You do not need to disclose or share any personal information you are uncomfortable with.

8. The final presentation is a closure with your character (for now). It is a way of gaining distance and separating. It is the last stage of the creative process when we validate and bring our creations out into the world.

9. Confidentiality—what happens in this *Final Presentation/Ritual* remains confidential. You may share your own process outside of the circle but not anyone else's process, words, disclosures, or creative expressions.

For the Therapist—Some Things to Reflect On

- How could knowledge about your own creative DNA be helpful clinically?
- How can you identify the creative DNA of those you work with?
- How could this process be used clinically, with what populations, and why?
- Are there populations that this process should not be used for? If so, why not?
- How do the stages of creative process relate to clinical practice?
- How and with whom could the use of a prolonged creative projection be an effective therapeutic tool?
- Did your experience of responding creatively affect your notion of the therapist/client dialogue, giving clinical feedback, and the role of the therapist?
- Did your experience of being a witness and being witnessed affect your notion of the witness role in therapy, and the experience of the client being witnessed?
- Did your experience of working individually within the context of a group process affect your notion of the role of a group process in therapy (if applicable)?
- How did working in a mythic framework affect you as a therapist? Did working with your character and story affect how you view therapy and your role?
- How did working with diverse creative mediums affect your notion of therapy?

CHAPTER 20

Afterwards

My character, La Loba, helps me to finish this book…when I doubt myself, she steps in to sing over the old bones of my past, reminding me that transformation is always possible… My words on the page are just the bones coming to life in a new way…

What happens after we finish the last step of the *Story Within* process? What do we do with the masks, the art work, our journals, and most importantly with the insights and wisdom we discovered? For some of you the process will continue maybe even for years, the relationship with your character deepening. While for others you may be finished and ready to say goodbye to your character for good. The experience of ending the process will be unique for each person. Only you can decide what this looks like. Here are a few questions to help as you find your way through the "Afterwards."

- What do you want to do with your mask? Put it in a container, have it displayed where you can see it, or destroy it? Make this a conscious decision. If you are not sure, keep it someplace until this becomes clear. Whatever you choose, before you place it or destroy it, thank it for helping you and find a way of honoring it.

- What do you want to do with all the creations you made (art work, soundscape recordings, writings)? You can find a box or container to hold it all, or you can get rid of some work and keep others. It is totally up to you, and remember, you do not have to decide everything all at once. The decision may evolve slowly over time.

- Notice for yourself if your character comes to you in your daily life. If so, when and how? If this happens, let your character continue to guide you and trust that it has more to teach you.

- If you are inspired, write down reflections about your process and send these to me via my website (www.yehuditsilverman.com). It would be wonderful to extend the circle of support to include everyone from all over the world going through the *Story Within* process.

Part III

ALUMNI WRITINGS

For 20 years I have been teaching a course in the Creative Arts Therapies Department of Concordia University in Montreal on *The Story Within—Myth and Fairy Tale in Therapy*. Throughout my academic career, from beginning as a part-time instructor, to full-time and tenured, and finally serving three years as Department Chair, this course was a touchstone, an essential reminder of what I love most. In every class, graduate students training to be therapists would leave their fears and academic books behind and enter their own unconscious and creativity. For many of them also it was a touchstone, a reminder of why they entered the field in the first place, and a way to reconnect with their own creative DNA. I was awed and often moved to tears by their courage to face their own demons and wounds and inspired by their ability to witness and support each other. I decided it might be helpful to include some writings from alumni who graciously offered to share their reflections on how taking the course affected them. Interestingly, and without planning, these pieces represent a wide span of time ranging from 2003 to 2017. They also demonstrate how different exercises and stages of the process affect each person in a unique way. Below are excerpts from each alumnus with a focus on what aspect of the class has stayed with them. And following are the longer and more detailed writings.

> "I took Yehudit's course about fifteen years ago and have been struck by how it stayed with me... Some of my best experiential learning happened when my comfort zones were stretched within a safe environment. As a teacher, I know how much goes into creating an atmosphere where experimentation, risk, and play can happen. It requires a lot, both in terms of facilitating and inviting learners, as well as not simply 'rescuing' those who are wrestling with or sitting in discomfort." Heather McLaughlin, ETA Lecturer, Art Therapist, Marriage and Family Therapist, Concordia University, Montreal, Canada (Class 2003)

> "I remember vividly how I left the Story Within course with a sense of satisfaction and fulfillment, feeling deeply connected with my authentic self, and astonished by the level of investment both emotionally and creatively that I had experienced. The guided structure of the process enabled me to take risks and explore deeply while working with my chosen character and my personal materials, served like a boat that carried me into the underwater caves of my soul... One of the many moments that stood out for me was when I created a life-size dwelling place of the character. With the mask on, I embodied the character and entered into her space. The exploration of the space was both textual and audible. I could literally feel how it was like living in her space. Without any particular expectations, I had a heart-to-heart conversation with my character that was almost like enlightenment to me." Chia-Wen Lin, Drama Therapist, Counseling Psychologist, Taipei, Taiwan (Class 2005)

> "The most memorable exercise was a painting that I created in which my main character had become two people, one trying to help the other... This painting allowed me to access my emotions in a safe manner by providing the distance that was needed to observe the interaction between these two parts of myself. I was able to capture my ambivalence between wanting to disavow my injured and vulnerable self, while at the same time wanting to rescue her from the

dark murky waters. Many years later, I was inspired to use elements of what I had learned in the *Story Within* course in my work as an Art Therapist." Erin Kuri, PhD(c), Art Therapist, Toronto, Canada (Class 2006)

"When I took the course, only one story highly moved me. It stirred up love, hate, disgust, sadness, and tears of anger. Nine years later, during my doctoral autoethnographic research creation, I was struck by the use of the same art materials I used in the course but in an amplified way… Also, directing other students to perform the scene of the wedding of the Princess helped me to step out from my perspective and to take distance from my fears to find a new way to deal with a relationship with a man at that moment." Mélissa Sokoloff, Art-thérapeute, Chargée de cours en art-thérapie, UQAT, Doctorante, Montreal (Class 2006)

"I am still in awe of how deeply powerful, inspiring, enriching, and moving this course was, and continues to be, in both my professional and personal life. I have been working in the field of drama therapy and play therapy with children, youth, and families for nearly 12 years. The *Story Within* process informs my clinical practice, with children as young as three years old, up to teenagers. It has been especially beneficial for youth who have resisted opening up in the therapeutic process, and for children who have experienced trauma, grief, and/or loss and can more easily explore their experiences through the world of another character and their story." Michelle Baer, Creative Arts Therapist/Play Therapist, Toronto, Canada (Class 2008)

"I made use of the story 'The Tale of Peter Rabbit' for my process… For me the book was associated with bedtime throughout my childhood in part. It also resonated heavily with me at a time in my adulthood when I was experiencing substantial grief-related sadness as it related to a resurfacing bout of a lifelong chronic illness… The framework of Peter Rabbit's journey fit viscerally with my own lived experience, triggering challenging childhood experience, yet containing it in a way that allowed it to be processed… As a result of completing this experience, I redirected my doctoral studies towards a comprehensive qualitative investigation of the grief of illness." Leah Lewis, PhD, Drama Therapist, Assistant Professor, Memorial University of Newfoundland and Labrador (Class 2010)

"The process lived in the *Story Within* class has affected me both professionally and personally…my understanding of the creative process and how to deal with traumatic experiences and grief was influenced by my experience in class. I believe that my character and my personal process within the group became fully activated and imbued with profound meanings because of the variety and fullness of the creative exploration." Connie Dancette-de Bresson, Lecturer, Universidad Finis Terrae, Santiago, Chile (Class 2014)

"It is a true testament to the process that, so many years later, I still think often about the character I chose during the course, 'The Story Within.' I remember feeling at the end of my presentation that I had opened a part of my story by telling Atalanta's and tapped into questions about what it meant to have those qualities and tendencies in me." Sonomi Tanaka, Art Therapist, Toronto, Canada (Class 2014)

"I also recall the final project—the culminating event—and how the journey of both Kai and myself intertwined… All the while I'm wearing my mask, my story became Kai's story and his story became mine. To put that on display, to dive deep within my own escapism and acknowledge it—let alone sit with it in confrontation—I feel really helped me to face it and learn how to change patterns of behaviour." Craig Flickinger, Drama Therapist, New York, USA (Class 2014)

"The *Story Within* class was perhaps the most profound experience during my two-year graduate period of becoming a therapist… Immersing myself in the story reflected a necessary re-engagement with my most authentic, vital creative force… This was a life-changing experience crystallized in a process that I can come back to with concrete art work, video, writing and find new meaning and reflections each time… The verification process, and in particular the performance in front of my class, is the performance I am most proud of in my life." Laurie Potter, Drama Therapist/Counselor, British Columbia, Canada (Class 2015)

"This course helped me in many ways and was the first step to help me feel like myself again, to remind me that my ability to connect with others is strong, if I can only get out of my own way. If I had not found a way to address this issue, I cannot confidently say that I would be the practitioner I am today, or at all. Having both the distance and the intimate nature that a story like this provides allowed me to immerse myself in the dark possibilities, the parts of myself that frighten me the most, before surfacing, and taking in that cleansing breath to know that that doesn't have to be me." Cayley McConaghy, Drama Therapist/Counselor, Edmonton, Canada (Class 2016)

"I continue to return to Persephone, years after participating in the *Story Within* process… Remembering Persephone gives me hope. During those periods when I live in my own private underworld, when I feel I can't move forward, she helps me seek the strength to find moments of light and purpose. When I feel disconnected from myself and my loved ones, she helps me to remember that there is another aspect of living that is full of love and connection." Alicia Winn, MA, Drama Therapist/Counselor, Toronto, Canada (Class 2016)

"For me, one of the most important moments in the process was the making of soundscapes. At first, the idea of creating sounds made me feel stressed and scared. I thought to myself, 'I can't make music, I can't keep a rhythm, what will people think…?' Despite feeling deeply uncomfortable, I started to hand instruments to my classmates and told them what to play. When I heard the group begin to play my soundscape, I was amazed at how touched I felt. It felt like something had unlocked in me, a new door was opening; I had found a new way to express myself." Anne-Laurence Mongrain, Art Therapist, Montreal, Canada (Class 2017)

Longer Reflections

Heather McLaughlin, MA, RMFT, ATR-BC, ATPQ, ETA
Lecturer, Art Therapy Practicum Coordinator, Art Therapist, Marriage and Family Therapist, Psychotherapist, Department of Creative Arts Therapies, Concordia University (Class 2003)

I took Yehudit's course about fifteen years ago and have been struck by how it stayed with me. It was my first class experience of combining movement, music, art, and drama, which for a person who only felt comfortable in the visual arts, was very intimidating to me. Thankfully, Yehudit ensured that the class experience respected our discomforts yet challenged us so that we could really stretch ourselves. What fascinating and rich experiences emerged in this unfamiliar zone! There was such a deep vividness to the experience as we engaged our senses to explore, grapple, and play with the myths and fairy tales.

I can easily bring experiences from this class to mind that hold so much complexity. These moments are still often useful as I consider my current roles of therapist, supervisor, and teacher as well as when I remember what it is like to be a student or client. For example, when we formed a drum circle it felt really uncomfortable for me. Because I felt like we were given genuine license to express ourselves however we wanted, it delighted me when I realized that—feeling true to the moment—I could silently drum. This was received with as much respect and welcome as anyone else's expression. While many group leaders might verbally convey a message that it is okay to express whatever you want, sometimes it can feel like non-verbal cues contradict that message. In Yehudit's course, the verbal and non-verbal messages were congruent, which felt powerful. Some of my best experiential learning happened when my comfort zones were stretched within a safe environment. As a teacher, I know how much goes into creating an atmosphere where experimentation, risk, and play can happen. It requires a lot, both in terms of facilitating and inviting learners, as well as not simply "rescuing" those who are wrestling with or sitting in discomfort.

When we were asked to choose a myth or fairy tale to guide our process, the myth that came to me was Demeter and Persephone. I wanted to explore my understanding of the relationship between conscious and unconscious landscapes, the intergenerational relationship along matriarchal lines, the ups and downs of emotions, and the life–death cycle. Researching this myth was fascinating. I found traces through history echoing this story: Innana/Ishtar, Salome, and Sleeping Beauty. Each story branched off into different landscapes and other themes that helped me deepen my engagement with my chosen themes. Although I made a mask in this class, I found that a mask I had made previously resonated more and so I brought it in to work with. It was a papier mâché mask I had made molding my own face and using very small pieces of rice paper. The process hearkened a death mask and the mask itself had an eeriness to it. However, it was in the form of a flower, which created an interesting tension. This mask spoke of some of the tensions that we were exploring in the class as we learned about the creative process: order and chaos, control and letting go. It still hangs on my wall.

During my training, I frequently heard the adage "Trust the process," which I now repeat as a lecturer and supervisor in the Creative Arts Therapies program. This adage became a meaningful, lived experience in the class. Inviting us to trust, however, required a safe base as well as sufficient direction and containment. From this base, it could be trusted that ideas would come. Movements would arise in ways that made sense. Nothing needed to be perfect. Any path could bring rich learning. Welcoming the unknown would be useful and playing along the edges of comfort would bring growth. These are core ideas in the creative arts therapies but we need to live these ideas in order to be authentically engaged when we encourage them in others. The myths and fairy tales gave us some well-traveled paths to visit that initially seemed familiar but transformed into something deeply and vibrantly personal. I think we each experienced some transformation en route and for this I am grateful.

Chia-Wen Lin, MA, Counseling Psychologist, Drama Therapist, Taipei, Taiwan (Class 2005)
I remember vividly how I left the *Story Within* course with a sense of satisfaction and fulfillment, feeling deeply connected with my authentic self, and astonished by the level of investment both emotionally and creatively that I had experienced. The guided structure of the process enabled me to take risks and explore deeply while working with my chosen character and my personal materials, served like a boat that carried me into the underwater caves of my soul. My character revealed to me throughout different stages of the process many aspects of her thoughts and feelings that were not accessible in the original text and demonstrated how she completed her journey of crossing-over, which led me to find my own strength and confidence to continue my own journey of crossing-over.

One of the many moments that stood out for me was when I created a life-size dwelling place of the character. With the mask on, I embodied the character and entered into her space. The exploration of the space was both textual and audible. I could literally feel how it was like living in her space. Without any particular expectations, I had a heart-to-heart conversation with my character that was almost like enlightenment to me. I encountered her subjectivity, and for the first time understood the story from her point of view.

This exploration did not stop after the course. After I moved back to Taipei, I had a chance to join other artists to hold an exhibition on the theme of "Finding Myself." Following my instinct, I created an installation of dozens of dolls that were all cocooned and hung up on the ceiling. Visitors were invited to make their own cocooned dolls and install them into the existing set. Back then, I knew it was a continuation of my process in the *Story Within* course, but I was not aware of the meaning until later. Upon reflection, I realize that what really intrigued me was the concept of metamorphosis, of how we would often die to our old self and come out with a new identity in many stages of our lives.

Inspired by this method, I started using some elements from the approach, mainly choosing a story and a character, creating a character mask and a guided creative process in some drama therapy groups. I found that using the framework of a story and a character as a starting point can easily engage the members in the following creative process. Based on the needs and themes of each group, I would choose some tasks from the original *Story Within* process and combined them with other dramatic enactments and creative techniques to facilitate the group. These groups were held mostly in community settings, schools, and some therapy programs.

Some members from these groups felt the need to continue their therapeutic process, therefore I invited them to form a long-term group to further explore the materials they discovered. Eventually, this group was able to develop its creative transformation materials into an open performance. They wrote and rewrote their scripts, played different roles in each other's stories, rehearsed and modified their contents and invited their friends and families to the performance. It was titled "Who Do You Want to Encounter Tonight?" We had three consecutive performances over a weekend in 2012. According to the audience feedback, many of them were deeply touched, inspired, and found the performers courageous. Real life transformations were also reported by the participants after the performance.

Erin Kuri, PhD(c), RP, CCC-S, OATR, McMaster University, School of Social Work/Gender Studies and Feminist Research, Toronto, Canada (Class 2006)
I came to the *Story Within* as an art therapy graduate student enrolled in Yehudit's course. Each component of the process was impactful in unique ways. I was surprised at how connected I immediately felt with the story that I discovered. Through the exploration of different characters, I was able to connect more empathically with different parts of myself, that existed at different times of my life, and for different purposes. I believe the character that I chose embodied interpersonal trauma that I had experienced in my childhood and adolescent years. The most memorable exercise was a painting that I created in which my main character had become two people, one trying to help the other (in spite of the shame surrounding the second figure's circumstances, symbolized by the figure's environment in the painting). This painting allowed me to access my emotions in a safe manner by providing the

distance that was needed to observe the interaction between these two parts of myself. I was able to capture my ambivalence between wanting to disavow my injured and vulnerable self, while at the same time wanting to rescue her from the dark murky waters. The realization at how strong this ambivalence was, and how this divide was impacting me in the present day, was both healing and empowering. With the awareness that I gained through the powerful processes embedded within this course, I was able to reintegrate parts of myself that had been fractured by the events I had endured so many years ago.

Many years later, I was inspired to use elements of what I had learned in the *Story Within* course in my work as an art therapist. At that time, I was working within a children's mental health agency that provided support services to young mothers, many of whom had also experienced different forms of interpersonal trauma in their lives. Upon Yehudit's recommendation, I drew on original forms of fairy tales that retained the complex situational and interpersonal tensions that the authors intended to illuminate. Within a closed group session, where cohesion had been built among group members, I read the story of Cinderella. I then asked the group participants to choose a part of the story that resonated most for them and to create a piece of visual art reflecting on this part of the story. Over the course of numerous groups, I was intrigued to see how many times my clients chose the scene in which Cinderella returns to the site of her mother's grave, a place of solace where Cinderella would go to cry. In the context of the attachment work that many of these clients and their infants were engaged in, I wondered about a connection between this scene and a desire to return to what John Bowlby refers to as "a secure base." Many of these clients verbally reflected on their art images and chosen scene as relating to their desire to have their own mothers present in their life, or sometimes reflecting on feelings of being emotionally abandoned by their mothers. For young women becoming mothers themselves, this is often an important time to feel connected with their own mothers. For many different reasons (interpersonal, sociopolitical, intergenerational trauma, etc.), many of these young women did not have their mothers in their lives, or their mothers were not viewed as safe or reliable sources of emotional support in times of distress. I believe that this exercise allowed these clients to gain the emotional distance needed to be able to reflect on their feelings of longing and disappointment toward their mothers (not always easy feelings to allow oneself to acknowledge when wanting to protect that relationship, particularly if the client was still dependent on the relationship). In a group setting they were able to see that they were not alone in their experiences of grieving what they needed from their mothers. Finally, the exercise offered self-awareness and empowerment with respect to how they may choose to create a different dynamic between themselves as mothers with their own children.

Mélissa Sokoloff, BScS, MA, ATPQ, Art-thérapeute professionnelle du Québec, Les Impatients Chargée de cours en art-thérapie, UQAT, Doctorante en sci. humaines appliquées, Univ. de Montréal (Class 2006)

When I took the course, only one story highly moved me. It stirred up love, hate, disgust, sadness, and tears of anger. Nine years later, during my doctoral autoethnographic research creation, I was struck by the use of the same art materials I used in the course but in an amplified way. They brought me back to the two masks I did in the class, to represent the two main characters, a queen and king. Why? What is the impact on my work as an art therapist?

It was the story of Griselidis, a shepherd that the prince married with the only condition that she would obey his will. After their wedding, the prince tested her virtue for instance in isolating her from social life, giving their baby daughter to another woman, and pretending that the princess had died. Griselidis was still obeying in treating him with love, friendship, and affection. The moment I chose in the story was when he rejected her from the kingdom and asked her to come back to prepare his wedding with another woman. This princess was, in fact, their daughter, but nobody was aware, except him. Since Griselidis succeeded in this last test, he explained the truth to the whole kingdom and changed the wedding into the one of the princess and her loved prince.

During the course, even if I felt very invested in the process of making the mask of the queen, I was surprisingly really distanced and not invested when I had to choose a costume. This detail has been very meaningful. The process of unrolling the papers of drawings made during the class brought back a childhood memory of seeing a woman on television forced by men to unveil her body so they could take photographs of her body without her consent. In the scene, her son of the same age as me, around five years old, was hidden and he witnessed what happened. During the creative process, I rolled up the papers because I was scared even to look at them. At home, the process of forcing the paper to unroll against the resistance, with the need to tape it onto the counter to take pictures, recalled this memory of this woman who was forced to open her dressing gown by two men who were grasping her arms while a third man was taking pictures of her. Through my mind as a child, I witnessed an abusive act of voyeurism on a woman. My first mask, made out of a copper sponge, didn't have eyes, nose, or mouth as if to protect from recalling this memory, or talking about it. The second mask for the king was made with a rectangular piece of hard plastic, opaque. The exterior side was covered with red velvet and the interior with metallic tape. It had only two holes for the eyes, no nose or mouth. When I wore this second mask, I let this emperor talk for the first time and I felt afraid to discover so much power, but then released to have found this inner authority figure and let it speak. It allowed me to accept the distance with a loved one and to trust something numinous larger than me, which was empowering and constructive. Also, directing other students to perform the scene of the wedding of the princess helped me to step out from my perspective and to take distance from my fears to find a new way to deal with a relationship with a man at that moment. The lightness of art performance in a safe group was helpful in that process.

Michelle Baer, MA, RP, CCC, Registered Psychotherapist, Creative Arts Therapy and Play Therapy, Child, Youth and Family Therapist, Toronto, Canada (Class 2008)

> Looking out from under a giant flower petal, slowly, cautiously, peeking out to see, is it safe out there? Can I come out and be

free? Am I too small to take on this world, or am I stronger than what I seem to be?

Reflections on "Thumbelina"

I am still in awe of how deeply powerful, inspiring, enriching, and moving this course was, and continues to be, in both my professional and personal life. In this reflection piece, I will share the ways in which the course has facilitated growth for myself and my clients, offering examples of the specific outcomes of the process in action.

I have been working in the field of drama therapy and play therapy with children, young people, and families for nearly 12 years. The *Story Within* process informs my clinical practice, with children as young as three years old, up to teenagers. It has been especially beneficial for young people who have resisted opening up in the therapeutic process, and for children who have experienced trauma, grief, and/or loss and can more easily explore their experiences through the world of another character and their story. The therapeutic distance of the story offers healing space, and the creative arts therapy activities, in combination with non-directive play therapy explorations that I have incorporated, allows complex connections to be made in conscious concrete ways, and on more unconscious levels. I have seen the most beautiful "aha" moments, and the most heartbreaking pain acknowledged, accepted, and released. One of these moments was a 13-year-old who was struggling with suicidal thoughts, anxiety, and months of insomnia. She selected the story of Sleeping Beauty, and initially did not see the connections. One session after embodying the mask she made, she suddenly realized she wished she could be Sleeping Beauty and felt like she had finally found peace in becoming this character. She explored, through a sandtray world, this peace, exploring what would happen if she were asleep, "as if dead," voicing that only then would she no longer feel the pain she was experiencing in her life. This opened up a conversation and a way into the pain, to allow us to dig into the source of this trauma via Sleeping Beauty's pain, and find new ways to heal.

I worked with Hans Christian Andersen's story, "Thumbelina." The story called to me after I struggled with selecting the "right" story.

This was all part of the process, of course, and the test of time has reaffirmed, over and over, how right it was. In March of this year, I was facing some difficult decisions, and Thumbelina popped into my mind. I ran over to the illustrated copy I keep on a display shelf, flipped through with my eyes closed and read the page that popped up, the moment where Thumbelina is edging out of the mole hole into the sunshine, about to be free, the image of the bird she nursed to health, offering her a flight to freedom to be herself, to spread her own wings. I thanked the book, the process, the journey that had led me to here, and easily, confidently made my decision, remembering that though I may be small, I am mighty indeed.

I am certain that the layers and possibilities of the *Story Within* process will continue to bring new discoveries in my personal and professional life. I am forever grateful for being a part of this journey, and hope many more will benefit from it in the future.

Leah Lewis, PhD, Assistant Professor, Counseling Psychology, Memorial University of Newfoundland and Labrador (Class 2010)
I took Yehudit's course on the *Story Within* during an early stage of my doctoral studies. I delved quite deeply into the process and found it to be in some ways transformational at a personal level. This input refers largely to the framework from the perspective of student-come-client, as I feel the core of my experience was therapeutic. I made use of the story "The Tale of Peter Rabbit" for my process. "The Tale of Peter Rabbit" is a widely known children's story by Beatrix Potter. Its origins are British and it is a story that is familiar to many, likely in association with childhood. For me the book was associated with bedtime throughout my childhood in part. It also resonated heavily with me at a time in my adulthood when I was experiencing substantial grief-related sadness as it related to a resurfacing bout of a lifelong chronic illness. My kidney transplant of 23 years had failed, and I was adjusting to hemodialysis treatments every other day. The physical adjustment was part of the experience, the limited freedom of a life-maintaining medical procedure, but the deep grief due to the health transition was likely more profound. I had entered

my studies at a juncture of uncertainty and was feeling disjointed in my research plan. My health issues were occupying a lot of space in my life and, in retrospect I realize, was impacting my ability to engage in any meaningful way with graduate school. I was navigating the challenge of finding a coherence within the context of health loss. For this contribution, I've reviewed my writing from my own *Story Within* process almost ten years ago. With the gift of hindsight, I now understand that not only was the experience therapeutic, but also transformative. It carried me from a grief-ridden chaotic response to illness. In my final paper, I reflect:

> My own journey too has been laced with experiences of chaos, namely themes involving lost control of the body, physical functioning being reliant on medical treatments, the attendance in which I have no say. I have to go, quite simply, or my body will cease to function. It is like an overly ordered chaos, producing resentment and generalized anger. My schedule is very ordered because of these treatments, yet within that exists a chaotic loss of control. The image of an ordered frame that encircles and contains the chaos surfaces here. It is a similar and recognizable containment seen in Peter's return home.

The process of the *Story Within* was applied to my lived experience via the contained aesthetic of Peter's journey, making its way slowly into my own conscious identity:

> The Tale of Peter Rabbit also connotes images of order and chaos. Peter's temporary loss of himself, launches him into a state of chaos; an experience that lacks order where confusion and desperateness is abundant. He is impetuous and rebellious, confused about reality. This, I perceive as a possible result of having no father. He opts to rebel towards the very place where his father was killed. The chaos within Peter, the confusion and grief of having no father, is externalized into careless, impish behavior.

The framework of Peter Rabbit's journey fit viscerally with my own lived experience, triggering challenging childhood experience, yet containing it in a way that allowed it to be processed:

His [Peter Rabbit's] mother notices this and worries aloud that he might be getting sick, so she tucks him into bed and gives him some chamomile tea to soothe him. It is such a warm, safe and comfortable image that affects me so strongly.

I have some notions, too, as to why I was so deeply affected by images of safety and comfort. As a child, early on, I spent a good deal of time at Toronto's Hospital for Sick Children. Living in Newfoundland in the 80s, these experiences were often spent without my parents because they were unable to get time off of work. Of course, such a scenario would likely proceed differently today, but somehow I feel that I longed for home (of course), but also my sense of safety and security became quite vulnerable. This is perhaps particularly poignant for me now because these issues have resurfaced recently with my health. I am a dialysis patient, having returned after a long (23-year) absence. It does not surprise me in the least that such childhood images are resurfacing for me as I revisit the very same vulnerable experiences I experienced then.

As a result of completing this experience, I redirected my doctoral studies towards a comprehensive qualitative investigation of the grief of illness. My engagement with the research was passionate and driven and produced a rich and evocative study that explored illness-related grief by layering the narrative of illness experience. I'm quite certain that this transition would not have taken place had it not been for my transformative experience contained within a therapeutic engagement with "The Tale of Peter Rabbit."

Connie Dancette-de Bresson, MA, Art Therapy, Lecturer, Magister Artes en la Salud y Arteterapia, Universidad Finis Terrae, Santiago, Chile (Class 2014)
The process lived in the *Story Within* class has affected me both professionally and personally. Although I have not used the method (because it is not appropriate for the population or context in which I work), my understanding of the creative process and how to deal with traumatic experiences and grief was influenced by my experience in class. The complexity of the creative process beyond

specific mediums and professional disciplines is something I try to communicate to my students. I believe that my character and my personal process within the group became fully activated and imbued with profound meanings because of the variety and fullness of the creative exploration. Through song and silence, needles and light, glares and footsteps, my character and his Helper became alive and able to guide and accompany me in my journey.

As I reread my journal notes and papers from the class, it is difficult to pinpoint specific exercises or moments in the process that stand out. I remember well certain moments (some magical and others painful) but more relevant to me is that my character and his Helper still *exist* in their essence and have lived on beyond the termination of the process per se. My Pied Piper feels as if he *is* a significant person so that despite physical distance, life circumstances, and time, the relationship somehow remains intact. As are those special friendships that are resilient to deterioration during long periods of silence and separateness and remain sacred. Mouse (my Helper) has literally not left my bedside table since I created him; Mouse is my cherished *adult* transitional object.

At a personal level, I feel a lasting effect from my *Story Within* process and it is impossible for me to lose track of time since it coincides with the year my son was born. I was pregnant during the class and, in so many ways, my physical, mental, and emotional preparation for my son's arrival overlapped with my in-depth exploration and re-enactment of my Pied Piper monster. It is here that I feel that I have things to say (or that at the time, they were left unsaid) as during most of the class and in my writing assignments, I never explored the role of my pregnancy or the undeniable presence and significance of my unborn child in the process.

It is evident for me today that my *Story Within* process took on the same intensity, chaos, and sensuality of my physical-emotional pregnant state. I was carrying a *real* child and also giving birth to and feeding my character. I was preparing a nursery to receive my child and constructing the world of Pied Piper and Mouse. I was ambivalent about having a second child and I needed to keep it secret for quite a while. Despite deeply desiring my child, I felt painfully aware of everything that could go wrong and overwhelmed by the extent of how my own personal baggage could weigh on my child.

It was with the urgency of my expected due date that I excavated into my character and his dark world. It sometimes felt like a freefall into darkness, impelled by unstoppable physical changes, with nothing to lose and with hopes of gaining lucidity and strength. The nature of my character of Pied Piper, one who lures, sequesters, and kills both rodents and children, seems like an ill-informed choice for a pregnant woman…and yet it was exactly what I needed. It is as if I needed to unravel everything, make a gigantic horrid mess, in order to reknit; I needed to create a monster (to be a monster) in order to create a child and become a mother. And it worked; I have become a better mother (and a better me).

In retrospect, I believe that my exploring the *Story Within* set in motion other meaningful steps beyond my relationship with my children. Shortly after my son was born, my mother and I began family counseling to work on our relationship and she then pursued other creative interventions of great significance in our family history and dynamics. In short, with Pied Piper, something shifted and everything else fell into a good-enough place.

Sonomi Tanaka, MA, RP, Art Therapist, Private Practice, Arterie, Toronto, Canada (Class 2014)
It is a true testament to the process that, so many years later, I still think often about the character I chose during the course "The Story Within." There are many moments from that course that stick out for me but I will narrow it down to two: embodying the mask in character and the final presentation.

I chose the mythological character Atalanta, and the unfurling of her story, as a focus for personal exploration in the course. During the creation of the mask representing Atalanta, I remember feeling as if the character was taking on a life of her own and that she was driving the creation of the mask, not myself. The character of Atalanta showed herself to be a very primal and rough character, as she was raised by bears. I wanted the materials used to represent her to resemble bone and fur and, because her later story involves her getting distracted by golden apples, I also included flecks of gold. In making the mask and wearing it, I understood for the first time the power of the mask in how it can embody a character that takes over when it is worn. When I look at the mask today, it still retains a presence, as if the character lives within it and stares back at me to remind me of who she was and what her story says about me.

The last presentation brought together pieces of who Atalanta was to me; fierce determination, constantly running, but also simultaneously facing her demons. I chose to make a stop animation using a light box, mylar and oil sticks. The materials were important for this as the light box gave a glow and ethereal softness, while the oil sticks on mylar gave a muddy organic feeling. I chose throat singing to accompany the piece and added my own breathing as the breath became an important driving force for the story. I remember feeling at the end of my presentation that I had opened a part of my story by telling Atalanta's and tapped into questions about what it meant to have those qualities and tendencies in me.

As a clinician I have used pieces of the process like mask making, storytelling and creating a life-sized space that can be explored. As a student in Yehudit's course, her process engaged me in a deep knowing through a journey, and I found that studying with her added valuable understanding of the use of metaphor and stories in healing and self-exploration.

Craig Flickinger, MA, RDT, LCAT, RiverSpring Health: Hebrew Home at Riverdale, Riverdale, New York, USA (Class 2014)
The character I chose for my mask was Kai from Hans Christian Andersen's "The Snow Queen." Upon reflection, I would say that the process was semi-challenging, if only because I was willing to go with the process and was also slightly trepidatious. This was during a period in my life when I had been confronted with all of the change that had occurred since I was a pre-teen, and it was illuminating to realize I've dealt with multiple levels of feeling lost. Some of these feelings included that of feeling lost in my burgeoning career, lost in defining my sexual identity, and the loss of my father in the 9/11 terrorist attacks and its after-effects many years later.

Regarding the process, I specifically recall the first time I put the mask on and had to inhabit the character. Within this story, the boy Kai is whisked away by the eponymous Snow Queen and he deals with feelings of being lost, trying to escape, and getting home. Most of my life I've engaged in some form of escapism, whether that be through theatre or distancing myself from my emotions, bottling them up and then having bouts of anger towards friends and family. I was very detached from my feelings and struggled with body issues as well. To have a contained space where I'm actively confronting those escape plans, those actions or inactions…it was both scary and exciting. I'm not sure if there was this instantaneous, complete sort of transmogrification, but it did occur as I wore the mask. The effects were not ephemeral, nor were they lingering after I de-roled.

I also recall the final project—the culminating event—and how the journey of both Kai and myself intertwined. Trauma has definitely lived on in my body and mind since age 11 and this experience was a purgation. I used a compilation of music to reflect my journey and how I've coped over the years. The music blended showtunes (specifically from *Next to Normal*, Disney's *Frozen*, and the TV series *Smash*) and bits and pieces of Tchaikovsky's *Swan Lake*, all of which had some form of lyrical desire for escape or stability. All the while I was wearing my mask, my story became Kai's story and his story became mine. To put that on display, to dive deep within my own escapism and acknowledge it—let alone sit with it in confrontation—I feel really helped me to face it and learn how to change patterns of behavior. Kai wanted to get home and I believe that ultimately, I've wanted those same feelings: of home, of belonging, of solid ground.

Laurie Potter, MA, Mental Health Counselor/Creative Arts Therapist, British Columbia, Canada (Class 2015)
The *Story Within* process was perhaps the most profound experience during my two-year graduate period of becoming a therapist. My encounter with "Alleleirauh" was during a time of necessary purgation, a ritual cleansing of someone or something. The story came to me during a period of deep psychological work in which I sought to free myself of a dominant father complex and bring

myself towards conscious femininity. I still admire my character's attempt to break from all the ideals of perfection projected onto her by covering herself in a mantle of fur and earth and taking off into the woods. Immersing myself in the story reflected a necessary re-engagement with my most authentic, vital creative force. This process mobilized my creative drive and revealed it to me as an innate impulse for healing. Coinciding with this birth of creativity and awareness was a simultaneous death; flowing tears of grief marked a huge psychological shift and period of individuation that I encountered. My adherence to patriarchal standards of perfectionism and being "not good enough" was so deeply entrenched that it was now self-imposed. I let an old story of the past die and it felt like a period of mourning. This was a life-changing experience crystallized in a process that I can come back to with concrete art work, video, writing and find new meaning and reflections each time.

The verification process, and in particular the performance in front of my class, is the performance I am most proud of in my life. I wanted to engage my body in an oscillation between free and bound flow to reflect the psychological chaos and order I had felt throughout the process. I explored what had been revealed to me throughout the myth and fairy tale process; I surrendered to exploring unresolved complexes, which dominated me, and faced it with readiness and vulnerability. This part of the process allowed me to bring together many findings from the journey. I examined the prominent archetypal energies before me, which spoke to me in dreams, authentic movement, literature and in my writing. All of this work culminated in the performance I feel most fully represents who I was and parts of who I continue to be. My performance sought not to deny fragmentation but to reveal it and embrace it. This was an incredibly validating aspect of the creative process and manifested in the freedom I felt to express authentically during my final presentation; the feeling of having to conform myself or attune my need to others to be loved had dissipated. Although I felt vulnerable, the group's empathic and observational stance provided a safe holding space for me to explore the unconscious depths of my character safely.

I use aspects of the creative process on a daily basis with clients but adapt the inquiry and exploration of a myth or fairy tale to different aspects of their life. We use projection to explore different parts of their struggles and this acts as a container for the journey into "not knowing." Using the creative process to investigate on a visual and sensory level usually leads to insights and new perspectives not yet experienced in our work together.

Cayley McConaghy, MA, Drama Therapist, CCC, Alberta Health Services, Edmonton, Canada (Class 2016, Assistant 2017)
For me the ability to use empathy and compassion to develop connections with a client is the touchstone of a good therapist. This is why I, at the end of my first year of my Master's in Drama Therapy, felt completely misplaced and out of my depth. I was convinced that my ability to connect with others had completely evaporated and I had no hope of ever becoming an effective practitioner. It was in this state of mind that I began the *Story Within* course.

The story I worked with was "Goolagaya and the White Dingo," a myth originating from Australian folklore. I dove head first in the immense darkness of this tale and focussed on Goolagaya, a woman who alienates herself from her community, unable to connect or develop meaningful relationships, and yet so desperate to do so. The pain derived from feeling so isolated when one just wants to belong hit me hard. I knew the pain of being so disconnected, and yet not understanding exactly why. Through my process I discovered that Goolagaya's biggest barrier was herself. Her inability to come to terms with this ruined not only her own life, but the lives of those around her as well. And although I was drawn to her for a reason, I also discovered that I did not have to follow in her footsteps. Where she could not find the missing touchstone to help her reconnect to herself, I began to see a glimmer. This course helped me in many ways and was the first step to help me feel like myself again, to remind me that my ability to connect with others is strong, if I can only get out of my own way.

If I had not found a way to address this issue I cannot confidently say that I would be the practitioner I am today, or at all. Having both the distance and the intimate nature that a story like this provides allowed me to immerse myself in the dark possibilities, the parts of myself that frighten me the most, before surfacing, and taking in that cleansing breath to know that that doesn't have to be me. This is a piece of folklore, and it is designed specifically to scare us, to warn us, and to guide us, which is exactly what it did for me.

The following year I became an assistant for the class. At times I found it easy to see parts of myself mirrored in the students as they were, literally, sitting where I had been the year before. I had to negotiate the delicate balance of allowing myself to be affected by what I was picking up, while not being completely consumed. To help me with this I leaned on a revelation that I'd had the previous year; drawing with pastels is immensely cathartic for me. Although visual arts were never my specialty, I often got hung up on doing it "right"; this is where the class encouraging me to explore as many artistic mediums as possible led me. Finding I needed a way to release what these mirrors were reflecting, I allowed the paper and swirling colors to help me feel and let go so I could continue to act as an apt assistant and witness for the class.

One of the most impactful moments throughout both years came when aiding one of the students who was having some difficulties. This student said to me, "I know there's no wrong answer, but how do I do it right?" They were feeling like everyone else in the class was developing deep connections with their stories and generally "getting it" but they felt they just…weren't. It had been discussed in class that everything was up to personal interpretation and there was no wrong answer, but they could tell, by seeing the other students' processes, that there must be a right answer. I responded with, "I think maybe there are multiple right answers." Perhaps due to my ability to witness the whole class and really see the variations of what was happening, it allowed me to see that the right answer is the thing that feels the most right to each individual student. It wasn't up to me or the professor to judge what they did or how much they were impacted, the right thing was for them to listen to themselves enough to go where they needed to go. This was a definite turning point for the student, but also strengthened my own views of right versus wrong. It has reinforced the client-centeredness of my therapeutic approach, and allowed me a freedom in knowing that even if I don't always understand what my client is doing or why, if they're following what's right for them then my job is just to provide the safety and connection to allow them to do this.

Alicia Winn, MA, Drama Therapy, CCC, Purple Carrots Drama Studio, Toronto, Canada (Class 2016)
I continue to return to Persephone, years after participating in the *Story Within* process. I chose the myth of Persephone and Hades quickly, after reading only a few myths. When I read it I had a physical sensation in my diaphragm that I recognized as emotional resonance, a deep empathy. The feeling was powerful, and I knew that somehow this was an important story for me. In the myth, Persephone (the maiden of spring) is kidnapped by Hades and taken as his prisoner to the underworld. She remains a prisoner there until her mother Demeter convinces Hades and Zeus to release her, on the condition that she return to the underworld for half of the year.

I had a similar "gut feeling" when I chose the "moment" that I would focus on. I imagined that first instant when Persephone learned that she could return home to earth, where there was life, family and growth. It was when I reflected on this choice that I began to realize that Persephone's journey was my own. This "mysterious" connection that I felt with this character suddenly seemed so obvious; her passage from the darkness of the underworld, to the light of earth in springtime and back again, mirrored my own seasonal journey from depression through to mania. As a person living with bipolar disorder, this cycle was deeply familiar.

When I made my "Life-Size Container" I draped richly colored fabric of burgundy and black from a high point on the studio wall and secured it to the floor. Inside I placed a quilt on the floor, and a chair draped in fabric. I felt strongly that I needed to make this home in the underworld comfortable and warm. I remember clearly putting on my mask, enrolling in Persephone's body-mind and spending time in my newly built shelter. My strong impulse during that exercise was that

I needed to remain engaged in activity, and find purpose there in my underworld home. I had brought from my apartment some precious stones, a journal and yarn, and I kept myself busy. Persephone would not let this darkness swallow her; she was determined not to remain fearful or absorb herself in despair. I imagined her spending her days walking slowly through the caves of the underworld, finding beautiful stones and placing them in her satchel. She would return to her home and examine the rocks, getting to know every facet and detail. She would document her thoughts and explorations in her journal, and use her yarn to repair her satchel.

This has been an extremely powerful image for me when moving through depressive episodes. Remembering Persephone gives me hope. During those periods when I live in my own private underworld, when I feel I can't move forward, she helps me seek the strength to find moments of light and purpose. When I feel disconnected from myself and my loved ones, she helps me to remember that there is another aspect of living that is full of love and connection. I remember Persephone's strength, the strength that surfaced from my own subconscious, and her determination to remain active, her trust that she could rise above her circumstances and make her own meaning in the darkness.

Anne-Laurence Mongrain, MA, Art Therapist, Montreal, Canada (Class 2017)
The whole process of creating through different mediums allowed me to dive deeply into a vulnerable part of myself. I feel that the creation of a character provided enough distance for that to be possible. Through using a projected character, I was able to let go of some of my own notions and explore ideas more freely. This approach helped me understand my own creative process in a more profound way.

For me, one of the most important moments in the process was the making of soundscapes. At first, the idea of creating sounds made me feel stressed and scared. I thought to myself, "I can't make music, I can't keep a rhythm, what will people think…?" Despite feeling deeply uncomfortable, I started to hand instruments to my classmates and told them what to play. When I heard the group begin to play my soundscape, I was amazed at how touched I felt. It felt like something had unlocked in me, a new door was opening; I had found a new way to express myself.

I continued experimenting with sounds throughout the different exercises. Music had become a tool for introspection, a way for me to express myself through sound and reflect on the emotions that were being played back to me. The soundscapes allowed me to connect to my character, and thus to myself, in a deep new way.

I think for me creating those soundscapes held an important lesson about the limits that we set for ourselves. It reminded me of how difficult it can be to let go of an old definition of oneself. At the same time, it also taught me about how being uncomfortable and taking risks can lead to amazing self-discoveries. The process of creating a character and exploring it through many artistic mediums has opened my eyes to new ways of thinking about the practice of art therapy, and my own personal journey.

Part IV

ADDITIONAL RESOURCES

For information on future workshops, trainings, supervision, and presentations: www.yehuditsilverman.com

Follow on Facebook: www.facebook.com/TheStoryWithinfilm; www.facebook.com/TheHiddenFaceOfSuicide

The Story Within
Film

The Story Within—Myth and Fairy Tale in Therapy © 2004

    Produced, written, and directed by Yehudit Silverman (53 minutes)

    Featuring Sonja Boudajee, Benedicte Deschamps, Patti Dray, David Jan, Gale Ostroff, Kalie Rae

    Original music composed by Yehudit Silverman, Jeffery May, and John Rundell

    Cinematographer: Martin Duckworth

    Sound: Glenn Hodgins

    Editor: Andre Elias

English with French subtitles

Six people embark on journeys of profound self-discovery by immersing themselves as characters in self-selected and personally meaningful myths or fairy tales. This film takes us through the stages of an original and dynamic approach to the creative arts therapies and is a moving testament to the power of creativity and myth in clinical practice.

DVD: www.yehuditsilverman.com

streaming access: www.reelhouse.org/yehuditsilverman/the-story-within

University Libraries: www.kanopy.com/category/supplier/yehudit-silverman

Publications

Silverman, Y. (2004). The story within—myth and fairy tale in therapy. *The Arts in Psychotherapy, 31*(3), 127–135.

Silverman, Y. (2006). Drama therapy with adolescent survivors of sexual abuse. In S. Brooke (ed.), *The use of creative arts therapies with sexual abuse survivors*. New York, NY: Charles C. Thomas.

Work Around the Issue of Suicide
Film

The Hidden Face of Suicide © March 2010

Produced, written, and directed by Yehudit Silverman (58 minutes)

Original music composed by Yehudit Silverman

Cinematographer: Martin Duckworth

Sound: Glenn Hodgins

Editor: Andre Elias

English with French subtitles, dubbed into Polish

Available from www.reelhouse.org/yehuditsilverman/the-hidden-face-of-suicide

And www.yehuditsilverman.com and University Libraries (www.kanopy.com/category/supplier/yehudit-silverman)

This film enters the world of survivors, those who have lost loved ones to suicide, and reveals their remarkable stories. Looking for the story behind the silence in her own family, Silverman sets out on a journey of understanding and transformation. Using masks, the survivors find a unique and creative way to express the unspeakable. Their journey brings to light the danger of secrets and the terrible cost of silence.

Publications

Silverman, Y. (2013). *We need to talk more not less about suicide.* Opinion piece, Montreal Gazette, May 7, 2013.

Silverman, Y. (2018). Choosing to enter the darkness—a researcher's reflection on working with suicide survivors: A collage of words and images. *Qualitative Research in Psychology.* https://doi.org/10.1080/14780887.2018.1442766

Silverman, Y., Smith, F., and Burns, M. (2013). Coming together in pain and joy: A multicultural and arts-based suicide awareness project. *The Arts in Psychotherapy, 40,* 216–223.

Seeds of Hope Project

Seeds of Hope: An arts-based approach to working with suicide and resiliency in collaboration with the Montreal Museum of Fine Arts. Participation from diverse communities including Inuit, survivors, attempters, and support workers in arts-based workshops making masks as means of expressing the pain, trauma, and hope around the issue.

Public exhibition at the Montreal Museum of Fine Arts March 8–April 3, 2017.

Funded by Concordia University and the Montreal Museum of Fine Arts 2015–2017.

Seeds of Hope Videos: *The Process* 9:07 © 2017, *The Images* 5:32 © 2017, in English and French.

Seeds of Hope website (English and French): https://seedsofhopemontreal.wixsite.com/seedsofhope; https://seedsofhopemontreal.wixsite.com/grainesdespoir

Creative Arts Therapies Organizations

"Creative Arts Therapies" is an umbrella term for healthcare professions that use creative mediums (art, music, drama, dance) to improve and enhance the psychological and social wellbeing of individuals of all ages and health conditions. Professional training involves a Master's degree from an accredited university (BA and/or MA for music therapy) plus many additional hours of supervised clinical work to become accredited.

For more information on professional training programs, therapists, conferences, etc., please contact the organizations listed below.

Australia

Australian, New Zealand and Asian Creative Arts Therapies Association (ANZACATA)

www.anzacata.org

Canada

Canadian Art Therapy Association or Association Canadienne d'Art Thérapie (CATA-ACAT)

www.canadianarttherapy.org

Canadian Association of Music Therapists (CAMT)

www.musictherapy.ca

Dance Movement Therapy Association in Canada (DMTAC)

www.dmtac.org

Quebec Chapter of NADTA

www.nadta.org/about-nadta/local-chapters/quebec-chapter.html

UK

Association for Dance Movement Psychotherapy UK (ADMP UK)

https://admp.org.uk

British Association for Music Therapy (BAMT)

www.bamt.org

British Association of Art Therapists (BAAT)

www.baat.org

British Association of Dramatherapists (BADth)

https://badth.org.uk

US

American Art Therapy Association (AATA)

https://arttherapy.org/about

American Dance Therapy Association (ADTA)

https://adta.org

American Music Therapy Association (AMTA)

www.musictherapy.org

National Coalition of Creative Arts Therapies Associations, Inc. (NCCATA)

www.nccata.org

North American Drama Therapy Association (NADTA)

www.nadta.org

References

Adler, J. (2002). *Offering from the conscious body: The discipline of authentic movement.* Rochester, NY: Inner Traditions.

Adler, J. (2015). The mandorla and the discipline of authentic movement. *Journal of Dance and Somatic Practices, 7*(2), 217–227.

Ajili, I., Mallem, M., and Didier, J.Y. (2018). Human motions and emotions recognition inspired by LMA qualities. *The Visual Computer*, 1–16.

Ali, A., Wolfert, S., Lam, I., and Rahman, T. (2018). Intersecting modes of aesthetic distance and mimetic induction in therapeutic process: Examining a drama-based treatment for military-related traumatic stress. *Drama Therapy Review, 4*(2), 153–165.

Baciu, A.M. (2017). Fairy tales revisited: Identity making and unmaking. *Journal of Romanian Literary Studies* (10), 899–908.

Bailey, S. (2007). Art as an initial approach to the treatment of sexual trauma. In S.L. Brooke (ed.), *The use of creative art therapies with sexual abuse survivors.* Springfield, IL: Charles C. Thomas.

Bettelheim, B. (2010). *The uses of enchantment: The meaning and importance of fairy tales.* New York, NY: Vintage Books Edition. (Original work published in 1976.)

Bieleninik, L., Geretsegger, M., Mossler, K., Assmus, J., *et al.* (2017). Effects of improvisational music therapy vs. enhanced standard care on symptom severity among children with autism spectrum disorder: The TIME-A randomized clinical trial. *Journal of the American Medical Association, 318*(6), 525–535.

Binder, M.J., Martin, J., and Schwind, J.K. (2018). Exploring mindfulness in teaching–learning scholarship through a reflective conversation. In N. Lemon and S. McDonough (eds), *Mindfulness in the academy: Practices and perspectives from scholars.* Singapore: Springer.

Blatner, A. (1997). Psychodrama: The state of the art. *The Arts in Psychotherapy, 24*, 23–30.

Bolen, J.S. (2002). *Goddesses in older women: Archetypes in women over fifty.* New York, NY: Harper Perennial.

Bolen, J.S. (2004). *Goddesses in every woman: Powerful archetypes in women's lives.* New York, NY: Quill.

Bolen, J.S. (2011). *Like a tree: How trees, women, and tree people can save the planet.* Newburyport, MA: Conari Press.

Bolen, J.S. (2014). *Artemis: The indomitable spirit in everywoman.* Newburyport, MA: Conari Press.

Bollas, C. (2017). *The shadow of the object: Psychoanalysis of the unthought known.* (Anniversary edition.) New York, NY: Columbia University Press.

Botella, M., Zenasni, F., and Lubart, T. (2018). What are the stages of the creative process? What visual art students are saying. *Frontiers of Psychology, 9*(2266).

Buber, M. (1937). *I and thou.* New York, NY: Charles Scribner's Sons.

Buber, M. (2004). *I and thou.* London, UK: Continuum International Publishing Group.

Caldwell, L. (2018). Clarifying the transitional object concept. *Psychoanalytic Dialogues, 28*(2), 144–150.

Cambridge Dictionary (2019) Cambridge Dictionary. Available at https://dictionary cambridge.org

Campbell, J. (2008). *The hero with a thousand faces* (Vol. 17). Novato, CA: New World Library.

Campbell, J. (2011). *Myths to live by.* Csorna, HU: Joseph Campbell Foundation.

Campbell, J. (2017). Bios and mythos. Retrieved from www.scribd.com/book/349071305/Bios-and-Mythos.

Casement, A. (2012). The shadow. In R.K. Papadopoulos (ed.), *The handbook of Jungian psychology: Theory, practice and applications.* London, UK: Routledge.

Chaiklin, S. and Wengrower, H. (eds), (2015). *The art and science of dance/movement therapy: Life is dance.* London, UK: Routledge.

Chamberlain, K., McGuigan, K., Anstiss, D., and Marshall, K. (2018). A change of view: Arts-based research and psychology. *Qualitative Research in Psychology, 15*(2–3), 131–139.

Chierchia, G. and Singer, T. (2017). The neuroscience of compassion and empathy and their link to prosocial motivation and behavior. In J.C. Dreher and L. Tremblay (eds), *Decision Neuroscience.* Cambridge, MA: Academic Press.

Cole, J. and Degen, B. (2001). *The magic school bus*. New York, NY: Scholastic Inc. (Original work published in 1994.)

Conrad, J. (2017). Flying home: Aestheticizing and Americanizing experiences of exile and migration in the Second World War as fairy tales of return and restoration. In S. Buttsworth and M. Abbenhuis (eds), *War, myths, and fairy tales*. Singapore: Palgrave Macmillan.

Corntassel, J. (2009). Indigenous storytelling, truth-telling, and community approaches to reconciliation. *ESC: English Studies in Canada, 35*(1), 137–159.

Costa, M.J. and Costa, P.S. (2016). Nurturing empathy and compassion: What might the neurosciences have to offer? *Medical Education, 50*(3), 281–282.

Csikszentmihalyi, M. (1990). Enjoyment and the quality of life. In *Flow: The psychology of optimal experience*. New York, NY: Harper and Row.

Csikszentmihalyi, M. (2015). *The systems model of creativity: The collected works of Mihaly Csikszentmihalyi*. Dordrecht, NL: Springer Publications.

Cummings, C., Singer, J., Hisaka, R., and Benuto, L.T. (2018). Compassion satisfaction to combat work-related burnout, vicarious trauma, and secondary traumatic stress. *Journal of Interpersonal Violence*, 1–16.

da Silva, F.V. (2017). Fairy-tale symbolism: An overview. Retrieved from https://oxfordre.com/literature/view/10.1093/acrefore/9780190201098.001.0001/acrefore-9780190201098-e-79.

David, S. (2017). On integrating Jungian and other theories. In R.S. Brown (ed.), *Re-encountering Jung: Analytical psychology and contemporary psychoanalysis*. New York, NY: Routledge.

Davidson, R. (n.d.). Robert Davidson: Eagle of the dawn artist Ltd [artist page]. Retrieved from https://www.robertdavidson.ca.

Dhungana, R.K. and Yamphu, I.M.R. (2016). Indigenous ways of knowing in Nepal: Exploring Indigenous research procedures in shamanism. *Journal of Indigenous Social Development, 5*(1), 38–55.

Donati, M. (2004). Beyond synchronicity: The worldview of Carl Gustav Jung and Wolfgang Pauli. *Journal of Analytical Psychology, 49*(5), 707–728.

Dunne, C. (2015). *Carl Jung: Wounded healer of the soul*. New York, NY: Watkins Media Limited.

Enns, V. (ed.), (2018). *Counseling insights: Practical strategies for helping others with anxiety, trauma, grief, and more*. Winnipeg, MB: ACHIEVE Publishing.

Estés, C.P. (2008). *Women who run with the wolves: Contacting the power of the wild woman*. London, UK: Rider.

Estés, C.P. (2010). *The dangerous old woman: Myths and stories of the wise woman archetype*. New York, NY: Sounds True.

Frydman, J.S. and Mayor, C. (2017). Trauma and early adolescent development: Case examples from a trauma-informed public health middle school program. *Children and Schools, 39*(4), 238–247.

Gilligan, S. and Dilts, R. (2009). *The hero's journey: A voyage of self-discovery*. Bancyfelin, UK: Crown House Publishing.

Gordon, R. (2018). *Dying and creating a search for meaning*. New York, NY: Routledge. (Original work published in 1978.)

Green, A. (2018). Winnicott at the start of the third millennium. In L. Caldwell (ed.), *Sex and sexuality: Winnicottian perspectives*. London, UK: Routledge.

Hartman, D. and Zimberoff, D. (2009). The hero's journey of self-transformation: Models of higher development from mythology. *Journal of Heart-Centered Therapies, 12*(2), 3.

Henson, A.M. and Fitzpatrick, M. (2016). Attachment, distancing, and the working alliance in drama therapy. *Drama Therapy Review, 2*(2), 239–255.

Jennings, S. (1990). Masking and unmasking: The interface of dramatherapy. In S. Jennings (ed.), *Drama therapy with families, groups and individuals*. London: Jessica Kingsley Publishers.

Jennings, S. (2018). Trauma work in play and drama therapy. In B. Huppertz (ed.), *Approaches to psychic trauma: Theory and practice*. Lanham, MD: Rowman and Littlefield Publishing Group, Inc.

Johnson, D.R. (2009). Developmental transformations towards the body as presence. In *Current approaches on drama therapy*. Springfield, IL: Charles C. Thomas.

Jones, P. (2007). *Drama as therapy. Volume 2: Clinical work and research into practice*. New York, NY: Routledge.

Jones, P. (2016). How do dramatherapists understand client change? A review of the "core processes" at work. In S. Jennings and C. Holmwood (eds), *Routledge international handbook of dramatherapy*. London, UK: Routledge.

Jung, C.G. (2014). *Four archetypes* (3rd edition), (R.F.C. Hull, Trans.). London, UK: Routledge. (Original work published in 1953.)

Jung, C.G. (2014). *The archetypes and the collective unconscious* (R.F.C. Hull, Trans.), S.H. Read, M. Fordham, and G. Adler (eds). London, UK: Routledge.

Kennedy, P. (Host), Bertrand, P. (Executive Producer), Greenland, E., Kendi, M., Norbert, A., Andre, G., and Mitchell, E. (Elders), (2009, October 26). *Stories of the ancestors: The legends of the Gwich'in* [CBC Legends Project: Ideas]. Northwest Territories: CBC Radio.

Knight, C. (2018). Trauma-informed supervision: Historical antecedents, current practice, and future directions. *The Clinical Supervisor*, 37(1), 7–37.

Laban, R. (1975). *Laban's principles of dance and movement notation*. Princeton, NJ: Princeton Book Company Publishers.

Landy, R. (1993). *Persona and performance: The meaning of role in drama therapy, and everyday life*. New York, NY: Guilford Press.

Landy, R.J. (ed.), (1996). The use of distancing in drama therapy. In *Essays in drama therapy: The double life*. London, UK: Jessica Kingsley Publishers.

Landy, R.J. (2010). Role theory and the role method of drama therapy. In D.R. Johnson and R. Emunah (eds), *Current approaches in drama therapy* (2nd edition). Springfield, IL: Charles C. Thomas.

Landy, R.J. (2017). The love and marriage of psychodrama and drama therapy. *The Journal of Psychodrama, Sociometry, and Group Psychotherapy*, 65(1), 33–40.

Leeming, D. (2005). *Jealous gods and chosen people: The mythology of the Middle East*. Oxford, UK: Oxford University Press.

Leeming, D.A. (2010). *Creation myths of the world: An encyclopedia* (2nd edition). Santa Barbara, CA: ABC-CLIO.

Leeming, D.A. (ed.), (2014). Culture heroes. In K. Madden, S. Marlan, and D.A. Leeming (eds), *Encyclopedia of psychology and religion*. Boston, MA: Springer.

Levin, F.M. (2018). Learning, transference, and the need to suspend belief. In F.M. Levin (ed.), *Psyche and brain: The biology of talking cures* (2nd edition). New York, NY: Routledge.

Lim, D. and DeSteno, D. (2016). Suffering and compassion: The links among adverse life experiences, empathy, compassion, and prosocial behavior. *Emotion*, 16(2), 175–182.

Little Bear, L. (2009). Naturalizing indigenous knowledge [synthesis paper for Canadian Council on Learning]. Retrieved from www.afn.ca/uploads/files/education/21._2009_july_ccl-alkc_leroy_littlebear_naturalizing_indigenous_knowledge-report.pdf.

Little Bear, L. (2013). An Elder explains Indigenous philosophy and Indigenous sovereignty. In S. Tomsons and L. Mayer (eds), *Philosophy and Aboriginal rights: Critical dialogues*. Don Mills, CA: Oxford University Press.

Malchiodi, C.A. (2011). *Handbook of art therapy* (2nd edition). New York, NY: Guilford Press.

Marks, P. (2017). Fairy tales, nightmares and fantasies. In *Terry Gilliam*. Manchester, UK: Manchester University Press.

May, R. (1994). *The courage to create* (6th edition). New York, NY: Norton. (Original work published in 1980.)

McNiff, S. (2012). Opportunities and challenges in art-based research. *Journal of Applied Arts and Health, 3*(1), 5–12.

McNiff, S. (2017). The open space of art-based research. In S.K. Levine and E.G. Levine (eds), *New developments in expressive arts therapy: The play of poiesis*. London, UK: Jessica Kingsley Publishers.

Meisner, S. and Longwell, D. (1987). *Sanford Meisner on acting*. New York, NY: Random House.

Meredith-Owen, W. (2011). Winnicott on Jung: Destruction, creativity and the unrepressed unconscious. *Journal of Analytical Psychology, 56*(1), 56–75.

Moss, R. (2012). *Dreaming the soul back home: Shamanic dreaming for healing and becoming whole*. Novato, CA: New World Library.

Murdock, M. (2016). The heroine's journey. In D.A. Leeming, K.W. Madden, and S. Marlan (eds), *Encyclopedia of psychology and religion* (2nd edition). Boston, MA: Springer.

Obomsawin, A. (Director), (2017). *Our people will be healed* [motion picture]. Canada: NFB. Retrieved from https://www.nfb.ca/film/our-people-will-be-healed.

Okri, B. (1996). *Birds of heaven: Essays*. London, UK: Phoenix House.

Packer, T. (2007). *The silent question: Meditating in the stillness of not-knowing*. Boston, MA: Shambhala Publications.

Ragan, K. (2009). What happened to the heroines in folktales? An analysis by gender of a multicultural sample of published folktales collected from storytellers. *Marvels and Tales, 23*(2), 227–247.

Ragan, K. (2010). Asymmetry in male and female storyteller priorities: An analysis by gender of a sample of published folk narratives collected from storytellers worldwide. *Politics and Culture*. Retrieved from https://politicsandculture.org/2010/04/28/asymmetry-in-male-and-female-storyteller-priorities-an-analysis-by-gender-of-a-sample-of-published-folk-narratives-collected-from-storytellers-worldwide.

Rice, H. (2019). Herb Rice [artist's page]. Retrieved from www.authenticindigenous.com/artists/herb-rice.

Salmon, G. (2018). "Once upon a time"; The symbolic meaning of fairy tales and their use in educational psychotherapy. In H. High (ed.), *Why can't I help this child to learn? Understanding emotional barriers to learning.* London, UK: Routledge.

Seppälä, E.M., Simon-Thomas, E., Brown, S.L., Worline, M.C., Cameron, C.D., and Doty, J.R. (eds), (2017). *The Oxford handbook of compassion science.* New York, NY: Oxford University Press.

Siegal, D.J. (2007). *The mindful brain—reflection and attunement in the cultivation of wellbeing.* New York, NY: W.W. Norton & Company.

Silverman, Y. (2004a). *The story within—myth and fairy tale in therapy.* Documentary film (53 min). DVD: www.yehuditsilverman.com; streaming access: https://www.reelhouse.org/yehuditsilverman/the-story-within.

Silverman, Y. (2004b). The story within—myth and fairy tale in therapy. *The Arts in Psychotherapy, 31*(3), 127–135.

Silverman, Y. (2006). Drama therapy with adolescent survivors of sexual abuse. In S. Brooke (ed.), *The use of creative arts therapies with sexual abuse survivors.* New York, NY: Charles C. Thomas.

Silverman, Y. (2010). *The hidden face of suicide.* Documentary film (58 min)—(French subtitles available. DVD: www.yehuditsilverman.com; streaming access: https://www.reelhouse.org/yehuditsilverman/the-hidden-face-of-suicide.

Silverman, Y. (2018). Choosing to enter the darkness—a researcher's reflection on working with suicide survivors: A collage of words and images. *Qualitative Research in Psychology.* https://doi.org/10.1080/14780887.2018.1442766

Silverman, Y., Smith, F., and Burns, M. (2013). Coming together in pain and joy: A multicultural and arts-based suicide awareness project. *The Arts in Psychotherapy, 40,* 216–223.

Smith, D.G. (2018). Religion and spirituality of Indigenous peoples in Canada. In *The Canadian Encyclopedia.* Retrieved from www.thecanadianencyclopedia.ca/en/article/religion-of-aboriginal-people.

Smith, J.E. (2016). Folk ontology and the moral standing of animals. *The Chautauqua Journal, 1*(1), 7.

Stanislavsky, C. (1961). *Creating a role.* New York, NY: Routledge, Chapman and Hall, Inc.

Stone, A. (2015, February). How art heals the wounds of war. *National Geographic.* Retrieved from https://news.nationalgeographic.com/news/2015/02/150213-art-therapy-mask-blast-force-trauma-psychology-war.

Tharp, T. (2003). Your creative DNA. In *The creative habit: Use it and learn it for life*. New York: NY: Simon and Schuster Paperbacks.

Vogler, C. (2007). *The writer's journey*. Studio City, CA: Michael Wiese Productions.

Waboose, J.B. and Deines, B. (2002). *Sky sisters*. Tonawanda, NY: Kids Can Press.

Weymann, E. (2018). *Soundscapes in hospitals—music therapy perspectives*. Conference proceedings at the 13th International Workshop on Computer Music and Audio Technology, Hsinchu City, Taiwan.

Winnicott, D.W. (2016). *The collected works of D.W. Winnicott*. New York, NY: Oxford University Press.

Yalom, I.D. (2005). *The theory and practice of group psychotherapy* (5th edition). New York, NY: Basic Books.

Subject Index

aesthetic distance 33–4
agendas
　in therapeutic frame 64–6
alumni writings 205–30
approaching the inmost cave
　as stage in hero's journey 87
art-to-art response
　in Finding and Telling a Story 125–6
　therapeutic frame 67–9
attitude
　in creative process 101–2
auditory perceptions
　in creative DNA 38

Baer, Michelle 207, 216–18
birth
　as archetypal theme 92–3

call to adventure
　as stage in hero's journey 83–4
Chaos and Order
　in creative process 50
　description of 114–16
　exercises for 116–18
　homework 119–20
　and working with clients 119
childhood interactions
　as archetypal theme 93
circle of support
　for creative process 50
　developing 96–8
compassion
　in therapeutic frame 59–61
conceptual perception
　in creative DNA 39

creative DNA
　discovery of 24, 27
　emergence 43
　external process 43
　focal lens 41
　internal focus 42–3
　perceptual categories in 37–40
　product/process 42
　structure 43
　time factors 41–2
　uniqueness of experiences 36–40
　and working with clients 43–4
creative process
　attitude in 101–2
　circle of support in 50, 96–8
　descriptions of 46–8
　documentation in 100–1
　illumination stage 51–2, 55
　immersion stage 50–1, 54
　incubation stage 51, 54–5
　not knowing in 100
　objects in 100–1
　preparation stage 48–50, 53
　rituals in 100
　studios 49, 99–100
　supplies for 49, 98–9
　therapeutic frame for 53–6, 67–9
　verification stage 52–3, 55–6
creative projection 30–2
creativity
　innate nature of 27
　own relationship to 10
crossing the first threshold
　as stage in hero's journey 85–6

245

Dancette-de Bresson, Connie 208, 220-2
death and resurrection
    as stage in hero's journey 90-1
descending
    as archetypal theme 94
Developmental Transformations 168
Directing Someone Else
    description of 168-9
    exercises for 170-2
    process of 173-4
    and working with clients 172-3
Direct Attention
    in therapeutic frame 75-7
documentation
    in creative process 100-1

Edge, The
    description of 184-7
    different meanings of 10-11
    exercises for 187-90
    process of 192-3
    and working with clients 190-2
emergence
    in creative DNA 43
emotions
    in creative DNA 38-9
empathy
    in therapeutic frame 59-61
Encounter, The
    in creative process 50, 107-8
    description of 105-6
    exercises for 108-11
    homework for 112-13
    stages in 106-7
    and working with clients 111-12
Environment
    description of 158-60
    exercises for 160-4
    process of 166
    and working with clients 164-5
environmental danger
    as archetypal theme 92-3
experiences
    uniqueness of 36-40
external process
    in creative DNA 43

fairy tales 80
Final Presentation/Ritual
    description of 196-7
    process of 198-200
    responses from 194-6
    therapeutic reflections 201
film for *Story Within* process 16
Finding the Moment
    in creative process 52
    description of 147-8
    exercises for 148-9
    and working with clients 149-50
Finding and Telling the Story
    in creative process 50
    description of 121-3
    exercises for 124-6
    process for 123, 128-9
    telling the story 124
    and working with clients 126-7
Flickinger, Craig 223-4
focal lens
    in creative DNA 41

Goddesses in Every Woman (Bolen) 81

heroes
    stages in journey 83-91

immersion
    as stage in creative process 50-1
    therapeutic frame for 54
imperfections
    in therapeutic frame 59-61
incubation
    as stage in creative process 51
    therapeutic frame for 54-5
illumination
    as stage in creative process 51-2
    therapeutic frame for 55
internal process
    in creative DNA 42-3
interpretations
    in therapeutic frame 64-6

kinesthetic perceptions
    in creative DNA 38
Kuri, Erin 206-7, 213-15

Lewis, Leah 207-8, 218-20
Lin, Chia-Wen 206

Subject Index

Making a Mask
  in creative process 50
  description of 130–3
  process of making 133–5, 137
  and working with clients 135–6
McConaghy, Cayley 209, 226–7
McLaughlin, Heather 206, 209–13
meditation
  as archetypal theme 93
meeting with someone/something
  as stage in hero's journey 84–5
Mongrain, Anne-Laurence 209, 229–30

not knowing
  in creative process 100

objects
  in creative process 100–1
  in Encounter exercise 108–11
Obstacle and Helper
  description of 175–7
  exercises for 177–80
  process of 182–3
  and working with clients 180–2
Open Attention
  in therapeutic frame 75–7
ordeal
  as stage in hero's journey 88
ordinary world
  as stage in hero's journey 83

perceptual categories 44–5
  in creative DNA 37–40
  questionnaire for finding
  and working with clients 40–1
Placing and Embodying the Mask
  in creative process 50
  description of 138–40
  homework 145
  process of 140–4, 145–6
  and working with clients 144–5
Potter, Laurie 208, 224–5
preparation
  as stage in creative process 48–50
  therapeutic frame for 53
product/process
  in creative DNA 42

questing
  as archetypal theme 94

refusal of the call
  as stage in hero's journey 84
resurrection
  as archetypal theme 92
return with elixir
  as stage in hero's journey 91
revelation, transformation
  as stage in hero's journey 88–9
rituals
  in creative process 100
road back
  as stage in hero's journey 89–90

safety
  in therapeutic frame 72–5
schedules
  for creative process 49
shapeshifters
  as archetypal theme 95
smell
  in creative DNA 39
Sokoloff, Mélissa 207, 215–16
Soundscape
  description of 151–3
  exercises for 153–5
  homework 156–7
  and working with clients 155–6
stories and myths
  archetypal themes 92–5
  emotional response to 21
  fairy tales 80
  heroes in 81–2, 83–91
  meaning in 19–20
  myths as sacred stories 79–80
  negative elements in 9
  and positive change 9–10
  quest in 21–2
  stages in hero's journey 83–91
  therapeutic frame 61–3
  therapeutic uses of 12–13, 20–2
  types of 78–9
  universal themes in 80–1

Story Within process
　after last step 202–3
　alumni writings on 205–30
　Chaos and Order 114–20
　description of 22–5
　Directing Someone Else 167–74
　The Edge 184–93
　Encounter 105–13
　Environment 158–66
　film for 16
　Final Presentation/Ritual 194–201
　Finding the Moment 147–50
　Finding and Telling a Story 121–9
　Making a Mask 130–7
　Obstacle and Helper 175–83
　Placing and Embodying
　　the Mask 138–46
　Soundscape 151–7
　stages in hero's journey 83, 84,
　　85, 86–7, 88, 89, 90–1
　therapeutic frame 58–9
structure
　in creative DNA 43
studios
　for creative process 49, 99–100
supplies
　for creative process 49, 98–9

tactile perceptions
　in creative DNA 38
Tanaka, Sonomi 208, 222–3
taste
　in creative DNA 39–40

therapeutic frame
　agendas in 64–6
　art-to-art response 67–9
　comfort with creative process 67–9
　compassion in 59–61
　in creative process 53–6
　Direct Attention 75–7
　empathy in 59–61
　imperfections in 59–61
　interpretations in 64–6
　Open Attention 75–7
　safety in 72–5
　Story Within approach 58–9
　as witness in 69–72
　working with stories and myths 61–3
time factors
　in creative DNA 41–2
trials and tribulations
　as stage in hero's journey 86–7
tricksters
　as archetypal theme 95

verification
　as stage in creative process 52–3
　therapeutic frame for 55–6
visual perceptions
　in creative DNA 37
Winn, Alicia 209, 227–9
witnessing
　in therapeutic frame 69–72
Women Who Run with the
　Wolves (Estés) 128

Author Index

Adler, J. 70
Ajili, I. 75
Ali, A. 33
Aristotle 30, 62

Baciu, A.M. 22
Bailey, S. 33, 132
Bettelheim, B. 21
Bieleninik, L. 152
Binder, M.J. 64
Blatner, A. 168
Bolen, J.S. 81
Bollas, C. 21
Botella, M. 48
Buber, M. 106
Burns, M. 132

Caldwell, L. 22
Cambridge Online Dictionary 46, 62
Campbell, J. 20, 24, 80–1, 82, 83
Casement, A. 21
Chamberlain, K. 31
Chierchia, G. 60
Cole, J. 67
Conrad, J. 21
Corntassel, J. 22
Costa, M.J. 60
Costa, P.S. 60
Csikszentmihalyi, M. 47
Cummings, C. 59

da Silva, F.V. 92
Davidson. R. 131
Degen, B. 67

Deines, B. 81
DeSteno, D. 59
Dhungana, R.K. 22, 73
Didier, J.Y. 75
Dilts, R. 24
Donati, M. 21
Dunne, C. 21

Enns, V. 31
Estés, C.P. 22, 128

Fitzpatrick, M. 33
Frydman, J.S. 33

Gilligan, S. 24
Gordon, R. 47
Green, A. 22

Hartman, D. 24
Henson, A.M. 33

Jennings, S. 31, 140
Johnson, D.R. 168
Jones, P. 30
Jung, C.G. 21

Kennedy, P. 81
Knight, C. 32

Landy, R. 33, 140
Leeming, D.A. 24
Levin, F.M. 64
Lim, D. 59

Little Bear, L. 80
Longwell, D. 140
Lubart, T. 48

Malchiodi, C.A. 30, 132
Mallem, M. 75
Marks, P. 21
Martin, J. 64
May, R. 25, 47, 105, 106
Mayor, C. 33
McNiff, S. 31
Meisner, S. 140
Meredith-Owen, W. 22
Merriam Webster Dictionary 79
Moss, R. 73
Murdock, M. 81

Obomsawin, A. 81
Okri, B. 22

Packer, T. 75
Picasso, P. 47–8

Ragan, K. 81
Rice, H. 131

Salmon, G. 80
Saltmarshe, E. 14

Schwind, J.K. 64
Seppälä, E.M. 60
Shelley, M. 116
Siegal, D.J. 64
Silverman, Y. 21, 132
Singer, T. 60
Smith, D.G. 80
Smith, J.E. 132
Sōjun, I. 64
Stanislavsky, C. 140
Stone, A. 139

Tharp, T. 24, 27, 36

Vogler, C. 82, 83

Waboose, J.B. 81
Weymann, E. 152
Wilde, O. 131
Winnicott, D.W. 22, 30
Woolf, V. 26

Yalom, I.D. 31
Yamphu, I.M.R. 22, 73

Zenasni, F. 48
Zimberoff, D. 24

Yehudit Silverman, M.A. R-DMT, RDT, is a Creative Arts Therapist, and former Chair of the Department of Creative Arts Therapies, Concordia University, Montreal. She created The Story Within method out of her clinical practice and has been teaching it to graduate students for over 20 years. An award-winning documentary filmmaker, (with a companion film of this approach) she has screened her films on television, cinemas, conferences, and universities. She received several federal and provincial grants to work on issues around suicide, and interfaith arts dialogue. She leads workshops, trainings, creative rituals, and presentations internationally.

www.yehuditsilverman.com